The Consciousness Blueprint

Longevity, Soul, and
Humanity's Next Evolution

Maria L. Ellis, BBA, MBA

Ellis Publishing House

Washington, DC, USA

First Edition Published: 2026

DISCLAIMER

Cover Design: Jennifer Stinson
Editing: Cory Hott.

CONTENTS

DEDICATION

To my granddaughter Maven Rose, my grandson Phoenix Stephen and to every soul who senses that life is meant to be more luminous, more intentional, more deeply felt, no matter the number of years lived or yet to come.

To those who long not only for time, but for wisdom that softens the heart for peace that steadies the breath, for purpose that awakens the spirit and for joy that feels like coming home to yourself.

To the brave ones who refuse to shrink before the challenges of life who choose growth over fear, love over limitation, truth over comfort and consciousness over mere endurance, you are the torchbearers of a new era of awakening.

To every reader who has ever felt the whisper of something greater moving beneath the surface of your day, a call, a yearning, a remembrance, this book is my offering to that quiet, holy longing within you.

May these pages remind you that you are not walking alone, that the Divine breathes through your story, that healing is possible, that the true measure of longevity is not counted in years, but in the depth of presence, love, and awareness you bring to your journey here on Earth.

May this work guide you gently, lift you when you falter and awaken the ancient wisdom that has always lived inside your soul.

With all my love and devotion,
Maria L. Ellis, BBA, MBA
Author • Teacher • Soul Traveler

FOREWORD

When I first encountered Maria L. Ellis's work, what struck me was not only her intellect or her extraordinary body of experience, but her coherence. There is a rare alignment in her – between wisdom and embodiment, success and soul, action and awareness – that cannot be taught from theory alone. It can only be lived.

The Consciousness Blueprint: Longevity, Soul, and Humanity's Next Evolution is not simply a book you read. It is a transmission. It carries the unmistakable energy of someone who has walked through achievement, challenge, loss, reinvention, and awakening – and emerged not hardened, but clearer. Not diminished, but expanded.

In my years of coaching leaders, entrepreneurs, and individuals at the highest levels of performance, I have learned one essential truth: success without consciousness is fragile, and longevity without alignment is hollow. Maria understands this at a cellular level. This book speaks directly to the moment we are living in – a moment when humanity is being asked not to grow faster, but to grow wiser.

What makes this work exceptional is that it does not pit science against spirituality, or ambition against presence. Instead, it weaves them together into a living blueprint for the next stage of human evolution – one in which nervous-system regulation, emotional maturity, purpose, and awareness become the foundation for health, leadership, and longevity.

Maria invites us to consider a deeper question than "How long will I live?" She asks, "How awake will I be while I'm here?" And more importantly, "What quality of consciousness am I contributing to the world through my choices, relationships, and way of being?"

This book is courageous in its refusal to offer shortcuts. It does not promise transcendence without responsibility or longevity without inner work. It calls the reader into participation – to notice how consciousness shapes biology, how presence shapes time, and how inner coherence shapes the future of humanity itself.

You will find wisdom here that is both ancient and urgently modern. You will find compassion without sentimentality, clarity without rigidity, and inspiration without illusion. Whether you are a seeker, a leader, a healer, or simply someone who knows there must be more to life than acceleration and accumulation, this book will meet you where you are – and gently invite you forward.

Maria L. Ellis is not offering answers to memorize. She is offering a way of seeing, living, and choosing that restores dignity to aging, meaning to success, and responsibility to consciousness.

I believe this book arrives exactly when it is needed.

Not because humanity has it all figured out – but because we are finally ready to ask better questions.

Heidi Lagumina | Master and Platinum Partner Coach
Robbins Research International, Inc

IN THE LIGHT OF GOD,
THE SOUL REMEMBER

Before your first breath was spoken into time,
God held your soul in His eternal hands and whispered,
"Go, beloved. Live. Learn. Become."
You came into this world as a spark of His radiance –
spirit wrapped in a human journey,
eternity learning to walk in time.
And though the world taught you to forget your
origins,
God walked beside you in every longing,
and placed truth inside the quiet chambers of your
heart.
For awakening is not discovery –
it is remembrance,
a soft returning to the divine spirit
etched within your soul before the stars were born.

PREFACE

I am writing this book at a moment when humanity is moving beyond survival-based thinking toward conscious, self-aware evolution, confronting the limits of technology, speed, and control without corresponding inner maturity, and beginning to recognize that consciousness itself shapes biology, health, aging, and society.

In that sense, the book stands at the edge between an old paradigm (fragmentation, fear, domination, urgency) and a new one (coherence, awareness, integration, stewardship). It speaks from that edge, not from a settled destination.

A threshold between what humanity has known and what it is beginning to remember. Between a world shaped primarily by survival, speed, and separation – and a future shaped by coherence, awareness, and conscious participation in life itself.

For much of human history, we have treated consciousness as secondary: a byproduct of biology, a philosophical curiosity, or a spiritual abstraction. Yet today, science, lived experience, and quiet inner knowing are converging to reveal something profoundly different. Consciousness is not an afterthought of evolution. It is its organizing intelligence.

This book is an invitation to pause long enough to feel that truth for yourself.

It does not ask you to adopt a belief system, follow a doctrine, or accept ideas on faith alone. Instead, it invites inquiry – gentle, grounded, and embodied. It asks you to notice how your inner world shapes your nervous system, your health, your relationships, your sense of time, and ultimately, your experience of aging and longevity.

At its heart, this book is about integration.

It brings together science and soul, biology and meaning, awareness and daily life – not as competing explanations, but as complementary dimensions of the same living intelligence. It suggests that longevity is not merely about extending years, nor awakening about transcending the body. Both are expressions of coherence: the alignment of mind, body, emotion, and consciousness within the larger field of life.

The chapters that follow explore consciousness not as an abstract concept, but as a lived experience – one that can be cultivated through breath, attention, presence, and relationship. They explore healing not as something imposed from the outside, but as something that unfolds when the internal environment becomes safe, coherent, and receptive. They explore the future of humanity not as a distant technological destiny, but as a choice made quietly, daily, within each nervous system and each moment of awareness.

This is not a book about becoming something other than human.

It is a book about remembering what it means to be human – fully, consciously, and responsibly.

If you read these pages slowly, allowing reflection rather than rushing for conclusions, you may notice something subtle shifting within you. A softening. A widening. A recognition. That is not coincidence. That is consciousness responding to itself.

May this book serve not as an answer, but as a companion.

Not as instruction, but as invitation.

Not as certainty, but as a doorway into deeper coherence with life.

The future this book gestures toward is not waiting somewhere ahead of you.

It is already here – breath by breath, choice by choice, awareness by awareness.

And you are already part of it.

Maria L. Ellis, BBA, MBA
Email: mellis@fsacap.com
Mobile: 973-216-4181

INTRODUCTION: CONSCIOUS LONGEVITY: HOW SOUL, SCIENCE, AND HIGHER AWARENESS SHAPE THE FUTURE OF HUMAN LIFE

"The universe is conscious, and you are one of its expressions."
— Maria L. Ellis

There comes a moment in every life when we pause long enough to sense a quiet truth rising within us: we are far more than physical beings trying to survive on a fragile planet.

We are souls – eternal, luminous, intelligent – temporarily housed in bodies that respond to the quality of our consciousness.

This book is written for every soul who has ever wondered, "Why am I here, and what am I becoming?"

It is for the seekers, the healers, the dreamers, and the brave hearts who refuse to accept that human life is limited to biology alone.

For those who sense – quietly, intuitively – that we are far more extraordinary than we have been taught to believe.

And especially for the ones who are awakening later in life and discovering that transformation has no age limit, no expiration, and no boundary.

I have spent decades studying longevity, wellness,

spirituality, and the human journey. I have written about purpose, seasons, identity, and the emotional landscapes we navigate on Earth. Yet, as I stand in the later chapters of my life, a revelation has become clearer than ever: Longevity is not only biological. It is conscious. It is energetic. It is spiritual.

We don't simply age because time passes. We age through stress, disconnection, fear, and living out of alignment with the soul. Conversely, we thrive when we live with clarity, purpose, peace, love, and awareness. We expand our vitality when we expand our consciousness.

New scientific research now confirms what ancient wisdom has taught all along: the body ages, but the soul does not.

And when the soul leads, the body follows with new levels of harmony, resilience, and possibility.

In this book, I explore the extraordinary intersection of three realms that are often treated separately but are, in truth, inseparable:

- The Soul: our eternal intelligence and divine spark
- Science: the biology, energy, and physics of human potential
- Higher Awareness: the expanded states of consciousness that shape our evolution

I am writing this book now because humanity is entering a new era. A shift is underway, quietly, steadily, and beautifully. We are awakening to the truth that consciousness is not something produced by the brain; it is the foundation of life itself. We are realizing that healing is not just chemical but vibrational. We are remembering that love is a frequency, not merely an emotion. We are learning that intuition is a form of intelligence. And we are rediscovering that the soul speaks a language older than time.

This awakening is not happening only in spiritual circles. It is emerging in neuroscience, longevity research, quantum physics, near-death studies, meditation science, the global wellness movement – and even in the exploration of intelligent life beyond Earth. As surprising as it may seem, all of these fields point to the same truth: humanity is evolving into a higher expression of itself.

I have been deeply inspired by thinkers and researchers who approach consciousness not simply as a philosophical idea but as a measurable force that influences human health, social systems, and our capacity for growth. Some of these perspectives suggest that civilizations – whether human or beyond – progress not only through technology but through increasing coherence, cooperation, and conscious awareness. These are qualities humanity is only beginning to intentionally cultivate.

Whether one interprets these ideas spiritually, scientifically, or metaphorically, the teaching remains profound: a species cannot evolve technologically until it evolves spiritually. A soul cannot thrive until it aligns with truth. A person cannot live long until they learn how to live fully. The teaching points to a single principle: evolution – whether personal or collective – moves from the inside out. When consciousness matures, what we build, how we live, and how long we thrive naturally follow.

Conscious longevity is about more than extending life. It is about expanding life.

It is about living with depth, clarity, purpose, beauty, and freedom.

This book is an invitation, a journey into the deeper forces that govern how we age, heal, connect, and awaken. It is for those who sense that life is more than the body. It is for those who desire to grow wiser, healthier, and more soul aligned. And it is for anyone who believes that our future as humanity depends on the shift happening within each of us today.

As you read these pages, I hope you feel not only informed but uplifted. Not only educated but expanded. Not only inspired but transformed. My wish is that this book becomes a companion for your soul and a blueprint for your highest, healthiest, and most awakened self.

I dedicate this book to you – the luminous being reading these words – for choosing growth over comfort, curiosity over fear, and evolution over stagnation.

May these pages affirm what your soul already knows: that you are timeless, divine, interconnected, and capable of far more than you have ever imagined.

And to my family who walk this life with me, who inspire my heart, and who remind me daily that love is the greatest force guiding every chapter of our earthly journey, this work carries your light within it always.

Welcome to the next chapter of your life. Welcome to the next chapter of human evolution.

Welcome to Conscious Longevity.

With all my love,
Maria L. Ellis, BBA, MBA
Author, Teacher, Soul Traveler

CHAPTER 1:
THE AWAKENING OF CONSCIOUS LONGEVITY

"The privilege of a lifetime is to become who you truly are."
— Carl Jung

Longevity has long been treated as a matter of biology – of cells, genes, and the mechanical processes that sustain the body across decades. But every era brings a moment when a familiar idea must be re-examined through a new lens, and in this moment of history, longevity is no longer merely a scientific pursuit. It is becoming a consciousness practice.

Conscious longevity is not defined by the length of a life alone, but by the depth of awareness with which that life is lived. It is the recognition that the quality of our internal environment – our perceptions, beliefs, emotional patterns, and states of presence – shapes the body as meaningfully as nutrition, movement, or medicine. The body does not march through time blindly. It listens, continuously, to the field of consciousness in which it resides.

This book begins with a simple but profound idea: **longevity is an inside job.**

Not because biology is unimportant, but because biology is responsive. The body is never separate from the mind that interprets experience or the soul that gives that experience meaning. When we live unconsciously – rushed, fragmented, reactive – our physiology mirrors that fragmentation. When we live with awareness, our biology reorganizes around coherence.

Science has already begun to reveal what wisdom traditions understood intuitively. Epigenetics shows that genes are not fixed destinies, but responsive environments shaped by perception, emotion, and meaning. Neuroplasticity shows that the brain continually rewires itself in response to attention. Studies of telomeres demonstrate that the way we think about stress influences cellular aging as directly as any external factor. Even the emerging research on heart-brain coherence reveals that emotional regulation does more than calm us – it stabilizes the entire physiological system. A responsive environment is one in which biology is continually listening and adjusting. How we interpret events, how long we remain in stress, how we recover emotionally, and whether we experience connection or isolation all shape the internal signals that guide gene expression, brain function, and cellular repair.

In this way, environment is not something that merely *happens to us* – it is something we are actively participating in creating, moment by moment.

Consciousness is not an abstract philosophical idea – it is a biological participant, a force that shapes the body at every level.

Yet conscious longevity is more than the convergence of science and spirituality. It is a **way of living** that brings them into relationship. It invites us to inhabit time differently, not as something that erodes us but as something we participate in. It calls us to notice the inner climate in which we spend our days. Do we live in chronic vigilance or quiet presence? Do we interpret life through fear or meaning? Do we move from fragmentation or coherence?

Most of us have been taught to extend lifespan by working harder, trying more supplements, adding more routines, or managing our bodies as if they were mechanical systems requiring endless tinkering. But conscious longevity begins with a shift in identity. The moment we stop relating to the body as a machine we must control – and begin relating to it as an intelligent partner – we unlock the deepest mechanisms of repair and renewal.

The body responds not only to what we do, but to how we live while doing it. When we replace self-criticism with inner respect, our physiology softens into cooperation. When we choose awareness in the midst of difficulty, we signal safety to our cells and invite restoration.

This chapter is an invitation – not to master every scientific principle, but to understand that you are participating in your longevity every moment, simply through how you inhabit your life. Conscious longevity is not a future technology or a distant ideal. It is the daily practice of aligning inner life and outer action so the body has the conditions it needs to thrive.

When we begin to live this way, time stops being an adversary. It becomes an ally – one that shapes us with wisdom rather than fear.

In the chapters ahead, we will explore the landscapes that make conscious longevity possible: presence, regulation, meaning, connection, emotional coherence, the intelligence of the soul, and the future of human evolution. But every exploration begins here – with the understanding that awakening is not an event. It is a relationship with life itself. And longevity is not merely how long that relationship lasts. It is how consciously it is lived.

A Mini-Practice: A Single Breath of Awareness

Before you continue reading, pause for a moment. Take a slow, conscious breath in through your nose, feeling your chest and abdomen expand. Exhale gently through your mouth. Notice the subtle shift in your body, the way your shoulders soften, or your mind becomes just a bit quieter. This single breath is the beginning of conscious longevity. It is not a theory; it is an experience. In this moment, you have already felt it.

A Collective Awakening

Across the world, millions of people – especially women in midlife and beyond – are living longer than any previous generation, yet few were prepared for the emotional, physical, and spiritual landscape of an extended lifespan. They learned how to be productive, responsible, and resilient, but they were not taught how to become conscious in the later seasons of life. Becoming conscious in the later seasons of life means shifting from **achievement-driven identity** to **purpose-driven presence**.

Many are navigating internal changes that feel invisible to those around them. Their identity shifts as children grow up and move on. Unexpected fears surface after a medical diagnosis. Familiar roles rooted in youth or professional identity begin to dissolve. Caregiving takes an emotional toll. They appear steady on the outside while feeling unmoored on the inside. And yet, beneath all of this, something new is emerging. This season of life is not only about decline; it is a time of discernment. It is not only about limitation; it is also about liberation. It is not solely about loss; it is about a profound reorientation of what matters.

People in this stage of life often ask themselves new questions. They wonder how to live with vitality even as their bodies change. They wonder how to support their emotional and spiritual well-being alongside their physical health. These questions are not signs of weakness. They are signs of awakening.

The Science of the Awakening Body

We are living at an extraordinary moment in human history. For the first time, modern science is beginning to confirm what wisdom traditions have whispered for centuries: that how we age is not determined solely by time, but by how consciously we relate to our bodies, emotions, beliefs, and experiences. Fields like epigenetics reveal that our genes are responsive and dynamic, shaped by environment, stress, nourishment, relationships, and even meaning. Neuroscience shows that the brain is capable of rewiring and renewing itself throughout life. Studies of telomeres suggest that emotional well-being can slow cellular aging.

These discoveries are not just scientific. They are invitations. They invite us to participate in the process of aging with awareness and agency, rather than resignation.

What Conscious Longevity Truly Means

In this context, consciousness simply means awareness combined with choice. It means developing the capacity to notice what restores you and what depletes you; how your breath changes when you feel anxious or at peace; how your energy rises or falls depending on the environments and relationships you inhabit; how unresolved emotions linger in your body; and how experiences of joy, curiosity, and gratitude can create lightness and ease.

Most people age unconsciously not because they wish to, but because they were never shown another way. They push through fatigue, suppress emotion, normalize stress, and live inside habitual patterns of thinking and reacting that gradually shape the physiology of aging. Conscious longevity offers a different path. It invites you to pause, to listen, to inquire: What is my body asking for now? What is my nervous system signaling? What emotional waters am I moving through each day? What meaning am I living into? What am I holding that no longer serves my life force?

This does not require perfection. It requires presence. It does not ask for dramatic change overnight. It begins with attention, with honesty, with turning toward your lived experience rather than away from it. When awareness enters the process of aging, a profound shift takes place. Aging begins to feel less like something that is happening to you and more like something you are participating in. Participation restores a sense of agency. Awareness restores choice. And choice restores vitality.

From this place, longevity becomes less about avoiding illness and more about cultivating coherence – the inner harmony between your biology, your emotions, your nervous system, your relationships, your thoughts, and your sense of purpose. A coherent system functions more efficiently. The immune system becomes more resilient. Inflammation quiets. Stress softens. Sleep deepens. Creativity returns. The body begins to repair itself more effectively.

Yet conscious longevity is not only about physiology. It is also deeply about meaning. Disconnection – particularly disconnection from purpose, truth, or authentic expression – can diminish vitality just as powerfully as disease. When life loses meaning, the body often follows. Conscious longevity restores meaning by returning you to deeper questions: Why am I still here? What wisdom has my life made possible? What is ready to be expressed through me now? In earlier seasons, meaning often comes from building. In later seasons, it often comes from becoming – from integrating experience, refining wisdom, and contributing from the depth of who you are.

A New Era of Possibility

Today, scientific breakthroughs and ancient wisdom traditions are converging in unprecedented ways. Artificial intelligence is personalizing healthcare. Regenerative medicine is restoring tissues. Wearable technologies are tracking biological rhythms. Meditation practices are entering medical settings. Breathwork is supporting nervous system regulation. Trauma research is bridging psychology and physiology. Compassion is being studied as a measurable health force. Presence itself is now recognized as a form of medicine.

Conscious longevity stands at the meeting point of these emerging developments. It is not futuristic in a mechanical sense; it is evolutionary in a human sense. It asks us to grow older without growing numb, to grow wiser without becoming rigid, and to become simpler without becoming smaller.

At its heart, conscious longevity is a relationship with life — an invitation to collaborate with your body rather than struggle against it, to honor your emotional life rather than suppress it, and to listen to your inner world with curiosity rather than judgment.

This approach does not deny mortality, nor does it promise immortality. What it offers is far more meaningful: a way to live each season of life with awareness, vitality, and inner coherence. Every person ages, but not everyone awakens as they age. This book is an invitation into that awakening. It does not ask you to become someone else. It asks you to become more fully who you already are.

You do not need answers to begin. Curiosity is enough. Willingness is enough. The quiet inner knowing that something deeper is possible is enough. Your inner life and your biological life are not separate stories; they are one continuous conversation. Conscious longevity teaches you how to listen to that conversation with clarity and compassion.

Whether consciousness is approached as a philosophy, a science, or a set of practices, it ultimately becomes an act of remembering — a personal reckoning with time, change, vulnerability, and possibility. In the chapter that follows, I step out of the role of guide and into that of a fellow traveler, sharing my own awakening to conscious longevity — the moment life asked me to listen differently and to see aging not as an ending but as an invitation into deeper truth. Chapter 2 is the story behind this book, the human doorway into everything that follows, beginning where all awakenings truly do: with a life that appears ordinary on the surface and a quiet revolution unfolding within.

Breathing Exercise: Awakening the Breath of Awareness

(Three to five minutes.)

This simple breathing practice is designed to gently shift your nervous system from stress into awareness and from urgency into presence. It prepares the body and mind for conscious longevity by restoring internal coherence.

Posture

Sit comfortably with your spine upright or lie down with your hands resting on your lower abdomen or heart. If possible, close your eyes.

Step 1: Arrival

Breathe naturally for a few moments. Notice the rhythm of your breath without trying to change it. Simply observe inhale… exhale… Let your body arrive fully in this moment.

Step 2: Conscious Inhale

Inhale slowly through your nose for a count of **four**. Feel the breath expand your belly first, then your chest.

Step 3: Gentle Pause

Hold the breath softly at the top for a count of **two**. No strain – just stillness.

Step 4: Slow Exhale

Exhale slowly through the mouth for a count of **six**, as if you are gently releasing tension from the body.

Step 5: Repeat

Repeat this cycle **six to ten times**: Inhale four, Hold two, Exhale six

With each exhale, feel your shoulders soften, your jaw relax, and your inner world grow quieter.

As you breathe, silently affirm, **"With each breath, I return to balance."**

When you feel complete, allow your breath to return to its natural rhythm.

Guided Meditation: Entering the Field of Conscious Longevity

(Eight to twelve minutes.)

This meditation introduces the felt experience of conscious longevity – where awareness, biology, and inner presence meet.

You may record this for audio use in the future if you wish.

Begin by settling your body. Let your eyes close gently.

Bring your attention to the weight of your body – how it is supported right now by the chair, the floor, the earth.

There is nothing to hold up. Nothing to prove. Nothing to fix. Only to *be here*.

Take a slow breath in through the nose… and a long, slow breath out through the mouth.

Again, inhale. Exhale. With every breath, feel yourself arriving more fully into this moment.

Now bring your awareness gently into the center of your chest – the area of the heart.

Imagine that each breath passes softly through this center.

With each inhale, you draw in calm. With each exhale, you release what is ready to soften.

Now allow the idea of **time** to gently loosen inside your mind. There is no age here. No past to measure. No future to chase.

Only this living moment. Bring awareness to your body as a field of intelligence.

Not as a machine, but as a living conversation.

Your cells are listening. Your nervous system is listening. Your breath is listening.

Silently, inwardly, offer these words to yourself, **"I am open to a new relationship with my life."**

Let those words land without effort.

Now imagine a soft, subtle light forming within the center of your chest.

Not bright. Not dramatic. Just warm. Steady. Alive.

With each inhale, the light gently expands. With each exhale, it settles and deepens.

This light represents your **inner awareness** – your

consciousness.

Now gently allow that light to travel through your body:

- Into the throat
- Into the shoulders
- Down the arms
- Through the torso
- Into the hips
- Down the legs
- Into the feet

Let your entire body be softly illuminated from the inside.

You are not pushing energy. You are simply allowing awareness to arrive everywhere you already are.

Now silently ask yourself – without forcing an answer, **"What is my body asking for now?"**

Do not search for words. Simply notice any sensation, emotion, image, or subtle knowing.

If no answer arises, that is perfectly fine. Listening itself is the practice.

Now gently place one hand on your heart and one on your abdomen if that feels comfortable. Feel the rhythm of your life under your hands.

Breath. Pulse. Presence.

Silently affirm:

- "My body is wise."
- "My breath restores me."
- "My awareness guides me."

Let each affirmation fall like a gentle bell inside your being.

Now imagine yourself standing at the beginning of a long, open path. This path is not made of fear or urgency. It is made of curiosity and trust.

You do not need to see the entire path. You only need to take the next conscious step.

Feel the quiet sense of readiness within you.

Stay here for several breaths. When you are ready, begin to deepen your breathing.

Wiggle your fingers and toes gently. And slowly, softly, open your eyes.

You have just practiced **conscious longevity**.

Reflection Prompts

You may wish to journal on one or more of the following before moving into Chapter 2:

- What did I notice during the breathing or meditation that surprised me?
- Where in my life do I feel most depleted right now?
- Where do I feel most alive?
- What might my body be asking of me in this season?
- What does "living consciously" mean to me today?

CHAPTER 2:
THE SOUL AND SCIENCE: EXPLORING THE NATURE OF CONSCIOUSNESS

"We are not human beings having a spiritual experience. We are spiritual beings having a human experience."
— Pierre Teilhard de Chardin

For much of my life, I believed that science explained the body and that the soul belonged to faith, intuition, or mystery – as if these two realms lived in separate universes that should never touch. I trusted data, measurement, and logic to guide my decisions, while my inner experiences remained quietly private and unnamed. Yet as I moved deeper into questions about aging, healing, and meaning, I reached a point where those two worlds could no longer remain apart. What began as a personal reckoning with my energy, fatigue, and curiosity gradually became a profound inquiry into consciousness itself – a place where science and soul did not compete but converged.

The Moment I Woke Up: When Awareness Became a Way of Living

Awakening does not always arrive in a dramatic moment or through crisis, revelation, or the turning of fate; sometimes it enters a life so quietly that only the body notices it first. My own awakening came this way, in a moment so ordinary it could have easily passed unnoticed, and only later did I understand that it marked the beginning of a new relationship with my mind, my body, and the deeper field of consciousness holding them both.

For many years, my life appeared steady, productive, and well-ordered. I carried responsibilities with the discipline and commitment that had shaped my entire adult life. I woke early, organized my days, supported those I loved, and kept pace with the demands of work and service. From the outside, everything looked balanced. Yet inside, something subtle was shifting.

My sleep was lighter. My thoughts felt more crowded. My emotions surfaced more quickly. And beneath all of it, there was a quiet exhaustion that I could not easily explain. Not the exhaustion that comes from lack of rest, but the kind that comes from being disconnected from oneself without realizing it.

For months, I ignored these signals. I told myself I simply needed to push through. That this was part of aging. That everyone felt this way. But the truth was simpler: I was living from my mind alone, while my body and intuition were patiently waiting for me to return.

The Ordinary Morning That Changed Everything

It happened on a calm Tuesday morning. I was sitting in my breakfast nook – a small sunlit corner of the kitchen where I liked to begin my day. The early light streamed through the window, landing in a soft gold line across the table. A warm mug of coffee sat beside me, untouched. The house was quiet except for the hum of the refrigerator and the gentle rotation of the ceiling fan overhead.

The month leading up to that morning had been unusually full. Appointments, deadlines, caretaking, and emotional labor accumulated into a constant hum beneath my awareness. My body kept pace even as my attention drifted elsewhere – breath shallow, shoulders tight, energy quietly depleted. Nothing dramatic had happened, yet something within me was beginning to fray, registering first not as a thought, but as a feeling I could no longer ignore. As I sat there staring at the coffee I no longer felt like drinking, a strange stillness came over me. It was not peaceful at first. It felt like everything inside me paused – the thoughts, the plans, the habitual rush toward the next task.

My breath sat high in my chest, shallow and tight. My jaw felt clenched. My shoulders were drawn upward as if preparing to defend against something invisible. For the first time in a long time, I actually felt the weight of my body.

And then, without effort, a clear realization surfaced: **I am living, but I am not fully inhabiting my life.**

I placed my hand over my heart – not as a technique, but instinctively, as if my body knew before my mind did what was needed. My breath deepened slightly. I felt warmth beneath my palm, a pulsing rhythm I had taken for granted for decades. I inhaled slowly, and something inside me softened.

My shoulders lowered. My mind quieted. The mental static that had followed me for weeks dissolved into a gentle spaciousness. I was present – not in the way one arrives at a destination, but in the way one finally returns home after being away without knowing it.

I felt coherence. Not as an idea, but as a physical truth.

The moment was simple, almost fragile, yet something irreversible happened. I crossed a threshold I had not known existed. My awareness settled fully into my body. My intuition rose to meet me. My nervous system – so accustomed to vigilance – relaxed in a way that felt both unfamiliar and natural. It was an awakening without spectacle. But it was awakening.

The Quiet Realization That Followed

In that sunlit corner of my kitchen, I realized how long

I had been living divided from myself. My body had been whispering to me for months, signaling imbalance through fatigue, discomfort, and subtle emotional heaviness. I had dismissed these signals as inconvenience or age. But they were not inconveniences. They were invitations.

My body was not resisting life. It was guiding me back into it. As I continued to breathe slowly, another realization emerged with clarity: **My body knew exactly what it needed. I had simply stopped listening.**

This knowing did not arrive with drama. It arrived with peace. I understood, perhaps for the first time, that my body was not a machine to be pushed or corrected. It was a living intelligence in relationship with me. This was the beginning of conscious longevity – not a theory, not a practice, but a lived experience of presence.

Learning to Trust the Inner Teacher

In the weeks that followed, I returned each morning to that small breakfast nook, placing my hand over my heart and breathing with gentle attention. I was astonished by how quickly my body responded to even a moment of deliberate presence.

My breath deepened. My thoughts slowed. My emotions settled. My clarity increased.

Science confirmed what my body already understood: the heart, the breath, and the brain synchronize when awareness enters the body. Stress hormones shift. Neural pathways reorganize. Healing becomes possible in the smallest moments. But at the time, I did not need the scientific explanation. I felt the truth in my cells. I had awakened not into a new belief, but into a new relationship – with myself, with my biology, with the field of consciousness that animates life. Awakening did not make my life easier. It made my life more real. And in that reality, I found a freedom I had never known.

A Shift in My Perception

A few weeks after that morning, I glanced at my reflection in the kitchen window as I carried my coffee to the table. I saw the familiar contours of my face – the signs of age, the history of laughter and struggle etched gently into my skin. And yet something was different.

I did not see fatigue. I did not see decline. I did not see the passing of time as loss.

I saw presence. I saw a woman who had finally come home to herself.

I saw a life preparing to unfold in a new, coherent way. That was the true beginning of conscious longevity – not the desire to extend life, but the desire to inhabit it fully. Everything that follows in this book begins here.

Mini Practice: Returning to Yourself in a Single Breath

This simple practice recreates the moment of awakening from that ordinary morning and invites you into your coherence, one breath at a time.

Sit wherever you are – at a table, in your living room, beside a window, or outdoors.

Place your hand gently over your heart.

Take a slow, unforced inhale through your nose. Feel your chest rise into your palm.

Let the exhale fall softly from your mouth.

Repeat this for several breaths. With each inhale, silently say: **"I return to myself."**

With each exhale, silently say: **"I release what is not mine to carry."**

Do this for one minute – or longer if it feels right. Notice the moment your breath deepens.

Notice the moment your body softens and you become present.

This is your doorway into conscious longevity. It opens every time you choose to enter.

The Rise of a New Human Consciousness

When I speak of a "new human consciousness," I am not referring to supernatural ability or spiritual hierarchy. I am referring to a simple but profound shift that many people are experiencing. More and more, we are beginning to live with awareness rather than automation.

Throughout human history, survival required speed, structure, and obedience to external systems. Emotional intelligence, nervous system health, and inner life were rarely valued. Productivity was praised; stillness was not. Sensitivity was dismissed as weakness, and intuition was ignored.

But something new is emerging. People are discovering that the inner and outer worlds cannot be separated without consequence. Burnout is not failure; it is information. The body is not an obstacle to achievement; it is a partner in consciousness. Meaning is not a luxury; it is a biological necessity.

The "new human" is not a different species. It is an ordinary human being operating from a new level of self-awareness.

People are beginning to ask deeper questions: How does my nervous system shape my health? How do my emotions live in my body? How does meaning influence my lifespan? How can I live longer without losing myself? These questions are the foundation from which conscious longevity grows.

What I Mean by Consciousness

In this book, when I speak of consciousness, I am not referring to abstract metaphysics or distant spiritual realms. I am speaking of something intimate and practical: the capacity to be aware of your inner and outer experience and to respond with choice rather than habit. Consciousness is the difference between reacting and responding, between surviving and participating, between existing and truly inhabiting your life.

You experience consciousness when you notice your

breath tightening during stress or when you pause before reacting in conflict. You feel it when you sense that your body is tired before it collapses or when you recognize that something in your life is no longer aligned before it becomes painful. Consciousness is not something you achieve; it is something you practice. And in the context of longevity, consciousness becomes a biological force. Awareness regulates stress. Stress regulates inflammation. Inflammation influences aging.

What I Mean by the Soul

The word *soul* can feel mysterious or religious, but in this book, I use it in a grounded way. The soul is not a doctrine or belief system; it is the inner continuity of your being — the part of you that experiences meaning, connection, and identity beyond roles, age, and circumstance. It is the presence within you that remains when roles fall away, when appearances change, and when accomplishments fade.

You sense the soul when you are moved by beauty, when truth resonates before logic explains it, when you feel drawn toward meaning, or when you know your life matters beyond productivity. In the framework of conscious longevity, the soul is not separate from the body; it is expressed through the body. The body becomes the vessel through which the soul experiences time. When the soul is ignored, the body often carries the burden. When the soul is honored, the body often responds with coherence.

Longevity, then, is not only about how long the body functions; it is about how fully the soul is allowed to participate in life across time.

Why Consciousness and Soul Matter for Longevity

If aging were purely mechanical, awareness would be irrelevant. But aging is not a mechanical process; it is relational and responsive. People do not age only because time passes. They age from chronic stress, unresolved grief, emotional suppression, loneliness, disconnection, and habitual urgency. Likewise, people often heal not only through medication but through safety, love, belonging, purpose, rest, and presence.

Consciousness and soul matter because they regulate the internal environment in which biology ages. When awareness increases, the stress response softens, emotional integration improves, sleep deepens, immune resilience strengthens, and coherence increases. When meaning returns, motivation stabilizes, energy lifts, and the future feels participatory again.

In this way, conscious longevity does not replace science – it completes it.

Breathing Exercise: Regulating the Inner Field

(Four to five minutes.)

This breathing practice supports nervous system regulation and emotional coherence – the biological foundation of conscious longevity.

Sit comfortably or lie down. Place one hand on your heart and one on your abdomen.

Inhale through your nose for **five counts**.
Exhale slowly through your mouth for **seven counts**.
Let the exhale be longer than the inhale.
Repeat this cycle **eight to ten times**.
With every exhale, silently release, **"I soften."**
With every inhale, silently receive, **"I allow."**
When complete, return to natural breathing.

Guided Meditation: Meeting the Soul Through Awareness

(Eight to ten minutes.)

Close your eyes gently. Bring attention to your breath. No effort. Just noticing.

Allow your awareness to move inward. Feel your body from the inside – not as a shape, but as sensation.

Now sense the space behind your thoughts. The quiet between thoughts. This silent awareness is not empty. It is presence.

Now ask quietly within, **"What part of me is aware right now?"**

Do not seek an answer in words. Simply notice the stillness that notices. That is the field of consciousness.

Now silently ask, **"What remains when I release my roles, my titles, my age?"**

Notice what feels continuous. That is the experience of the soul – not as belief, but as presence. Remain here for several breaths. When ready, gently return to the room.

Reflection Prompts

You may journal on any of the following:

- How did I subconsciously view the second half of life before today?
- What fears about aging do I carry quietly?
- What feels alive inside me despite physical or emotional change?
- How do I currently define consciousness in my words?
- When have I felt the quiet presence of my soul without using that word?

Awareness is the beginning, but awareness alone does not change the body. The body listens most deeply to the **nervous system**, the bridge between mind, emotion, and biology.

In the next chapter, we move from inner awareness into the biology of regulation. We explore how stress, safety, and emotional coherence shape the aging process at the cellular level and how the nervous system becomes one of the most powerful gateways to conscious longevity.

CHAPTER 3:
THE UNIVERSAL FIELD: WHERE SCIENCE MEETS SPIRIT AND CONSCIOUSNESS BECOMES REALITY

*"A human being is a part of the whole, called by us the Universe…
a part limited in time and space."*
— Albert Einstein

For most of human history, science and spirit have stood across from one another like distant relatives, aware of each other yet hesitant to fully embrace. Science sought measurable proof. Spirit trusted direct knowing. One examined the outer universe; the other explored the inner universe. For centuries, these two ways of understanding reality appeared to belong to separate worlds.

The Moment the Universe Became Personal

There are experiences that arrive without warning, altering the shape of a life not through drama, but through a single, undeniable shift in perception. For me, one such moment arrived on an otherwise ordinary evening – a dimly lit room, a soft breeze moving against the windows. Nothing about the world around me suggested that anything unusual was about to unfold. But within me, something unexpected opened.

I was sitting on my couch with a cup of tea cooling in my hands. My thoughts were neither heavy nor hopeful; they hovered somewhere in the middle, like faint clouds drifting across an ordinary sky. I closed my eyes for a moment – not to meditate, not to search for meaning, but simply to rest. And in that small pause, something extraordinary happened.

The silence inside me expanded.

It stretched beyond the edges of my body, beyond the familiar rhythm of my breath, until it felt as if I were dissolving into a vast stillness I had never consciously felt before. My mind did not race, nor did it try to interpret what was happening. Everything became impossibly quiet. And in that quiet, a truth revealed itself with astonishing clarity: **I was not separate from the Universe.**

It was not a thought. It was not a metaphor. It was a sensation that filled me with a tenderness I cannot fully describe. The boundary I had always assumed existed between myself and everything else simply softened. I felt myself as part of something immense and intelligent, not floating within it, but belonging to it, woven into its fabric as naturally as starlight is woven into the night sky.

In that moment, my life did not feel small. It felt continuous. I understood, without needing words, that awareness is not confined to the body that carries it. The Universe was not something outside me. It was something I was participating in with every breath.

I opened my eyes slowly. The room looked the same, yet nothing felt the same. The ordinary had become luminous, not because it changed, but because I had. The quiet around me seemed alive. Even the air felt conscious.

That night, a profound companionship settled into my life. I no longer felt as though I were navigating the world alone. I sensed that I was held – supported by an intelligence that was not distant or abstract, but deeply intimate. It was as though something had always been whispering to me, and I had finally grown still enough to hear it.

What Changed after That Night

In the days that followed, I did not float through life in a cloud of mysticism. I still cooked. I still worked. I still worried at times. Life continued – but my relationship with it had fundamentally shifted.

I moved more slowly, not because I was tired, but because I felt connected. I breathed differently, with a softness that surprised me. I noticed small things I had overlooked for years: the way sunlight touched the table in the morning, the warmth of water on my hands. Everything seemed to hum with quiet intelligence.

And within me, something essential began to realign.

I realized how many years I had spent trying to manage life, as though I stood outside of it, directing, striving, pushing. I thought my mind had to control everything for life to "work." But now I sensed that life was not something to control. It was something to collaborate with.

This shift did not erase difficulty, but it transformed how difficulty felt. Instead of interpreting challenges as evidence that life was against me, I saw them as invitations, doorways into deeper awareness, deeper coherence, deeper truth.

A New Understanding of Healing

In that expanded state of belonging, a clearer understanding of healing also began to form. I saw that healing was not only physical repair. It was alignment – an inner coherence that allowed the body, mind, and soul to move in the same direction. I sensed, without fully grasping the science yet, that when I felt connected to something larger, my body responded as though it had been relieved of a great burden.

That night offered the first glimpse of a truth that later chapters will explore more fully. **Healing is a shift in relationship – to oneself, to experience, and to the field of life itself.** It is not achieved through force. It is allowed through coherence.

I did not analyze this at the time. I simply felt it.

Something in me softened, and my body softened with it. Something in me trusted, and my nervous system responded. Something in me rested, and that rest reached into places of tension I had carried for decades.

The science behind this – epigenetics, emotional regulation, the heart's electromagnetic field, and the quantum dimensions of healing – would become clearer to me later. At the time, I simply sensed that healing unfolded more naturally when I no longer felt alone in the universe. When healing is described as having a **quantum nature**, it does not mean something mystical or abstract. It refers to the understanding that at the most fundamental level, the body is not made of solid matter, but of **energy, information, and relationship**. Quantum science shows that particles communicate, influence one another across distance, and respond to observation and coherence rather than force alone.

Meaning Became the Anchor

Before that night, meaning often felt like something I had to create or chase. After that night, meaning felt like something already present, waiting to be recognized.

I realized that meaning is not something life gives us – it is something that arises when we meet life with awareness. Once I felt myself as part of a larger field of intelligence, every moment, even the difficult ones, carried a quiet invitation toward growth. That recognition changed the entire emotional climate of my life.

I became more patient with myself, more compassionate with my past, and more trusting of my future. This tenderness became a form of longevity in itself – a softening that allowed my body and mind to settle into coherence. Tenderness extends life because it **changes the internal conditions in which the body must** operate. When a person becomes more patient, compassionate, and trusting – especially toward themselves – the nervous system receives signals of safety rather than threat. This shift alone has profound biological consequences.

Self-directed tenderness reduces chronic stress activation, lowering cortisol and calming inflammatory pathways that accelerate aging. The heart rhythm becomes more coherent, breathing deepens, and the body moves out of constant vigilance and into repair. Over time, this state supports immune resilience, hormonal balance, and cellular maintenance – the quiet foundations of longevity.

Tenderness also restores relationships: with the past, by releasing self-judgment; with the present, by allowing rest and presence; and with the future, by reducing fear-based anticipation. This emotional softening conserves energy that would otherwise be spent resisting, bracing, or proving. What remains is coherence – a state in which mind and body are aligned rather than at odds.

In this way, tenderness is not merely an emotional quality but a **physiological strategy for** longevity. It creates the conditions in which healing becomes sustainable, and life can extend not just in years, but in depth, ease, and vitality.

Presence Became a Form of Strength

That evening taught me that presence is not passive. Presence is powerful. It is the strength that arises when fear no longer narrows perception and when urgency no longer drives the nervous system.

Presence became my new posture – not an achievement, but a way of inhabiting my days. Even now, when I touch moments of stress or uncertainty, I return to that night, that stillness, that feeling of belonging. It reminds me that life is not asking me to brace myself against it. It is asking me to participate.

Mini Practice I: Resting in the Field

Sit comfortably and close your eyes. Place your hand over your heart and breathe slowly for a few cycles. As you inhale, feel your chest expand gently.

As you exhale, allow your awareness to widen – not

outward, but inward.

Sense the space within your body, then the space around your body. Let the edges between the two soften. Do not try to feel anything specific. Simply rest.

Silently affirm: ***I am held within the field of life. I am part of the intelligence that surrounds me.***

Stay here for one more slow breath, then open your eyes gently.

Mini Practice II: Sensing the Field around You

If you wish, pause for a few moments and sit as you are. Allow your eyes to soften or close. Bring your attention first to the weight of your body, to contact with the chair or surface beneath you. Notice your breath arriving and leaving.

Now gently expand your awareness outward. Sense the space just around your body, as if you could feel the air embracing you. Imagine that this space is not empty but quietly alive. You do not need to visualize anything specific. Simply allow the possibility that you are being held within something larger than your thoughts. For a few breaths, rest as both a body and a presence in space – an expression within a greater field.

When you are ready, return to the words on the page, carrying with you even a subtle sense of being supported.

One afternoon, weeks after that first experience, I was resting with my hand on my heart. I became aware of a subtle tension in my chest that I had not truly noticed before. Instead of reacting with worry, I breathed gently into the sensation and silently said, "You are safe." As I continued breathing, a surprising warmth spread through my chest. The tension softened. My breath deepened without effort.

That moment changed how I understood healing. I had long believed that healing was driven primarily by doing – by appointments, treatments, protocols, and corrections. Now, I was discovering that sometimes healing begins with alignment instead of action, with coherence instead of control.

The more I paid attention, the more I saw that my body responded immediately to the quality of my inner world. When I lived in sustained stress, my energy contracted. When I lived in presence, my energy expanded. When I rushed, my body resisted. When I softened, my body softened too.

Each observation made the same truth clearer. I was not merely acting upon my body from the outside. I was participating in a field that was continuously organizing me from the inside.

This changed how I experienced aging. Time no longer felt like an enemy steadily stealing from me. It felt like a process. I was traveling through with consciousness. I was not simply growing older; I was being continuously reorganized by the intelligence of life.

One night, standing outside beneath a sky filled with stars, that understanding deepened. I felt very small – but not insignificant. I felt small the way a single wave feels small in comparison to the ocean, yet inseparable from it. I recognized that my life was not happening *against* the universe. It was happening *with* it.

That recognition softened my fear in a way no abstract reassurance ever had. I no longer felt as though I was navigating life alone within a silent, indifferent cosmos. I felt accompanied by intelligence itself.

From that point on, intention became very different for me. It was no longer just a mental exercise or hopeful wish. It became a way of entering into dialogue with the field of life. When I held an intention with clarity and calm, I felt something subtle respond. My nervous system steadied. My thinking cleared. My body relaxed into cooperation.

I stopped trying to "fix" myself so aggressively. I began to explore what it meant to align. That alignment became its own medicine. Even in moments of challenge, when fear or discomfort appeared, I felt less alone inside them. I felt held within something larger than circumstances, something that was not rushing me, judging me, or abandoning me.

This did not make life effortless. But it made life more trustworthy. And trust changes everything.

Today, when I encounter uncertainty, I do not immediately reach for control. I pause. I breathe. I listen inwardly. I allow myself to sense the field that is always present beneath the noise of thought. Instead of asking only, "What should I do?" I also ask, "How can I become coherent with what is asking to unfold?" That question has guided me more wisely than force ever did.

I now understand that healing, longevity, and transformation do not occur in opposition to reality. They unfold through partnership with it. I am not manipulating the universe. I am learning how to receive from it. In that partnership, my body has become wiser, not weaker. My energy has become steadier, not smaller. My sense of life has become gentler, not diminished. I do not mean that it has grown smaller or less meaningful. I mean that it no longer relies on urgency, force, or self-pressure to feel alive. Gentleness reflects a shift from striving to attunement — from pushing against life to moving in rhythm with it.

I am no longer trying to outrun time. I am learning how to move with the field that carries time itself. In that movement, I no longer feel like a separate being struggling to survive in a vast universe. I feel like a conscious expression of a universe that has always known how to sustain life.

The Field beneath All Things

At the smallest measurable levels of existence, scientists have uncovered findings that challenge classical views of matter. What appears solid is largely empty space, and beneath the atom, subatomic particles do not behave like miniature objects moving predictably through space. Instead, they are described as probability waves — patterns of potential that take measurable form only when observed or interacted with.

This means that the physical world is not the deepest level of reality. Energy is deeper. Information is deeper.

Consciousness is deeper. Spirit has always taught this. Science is now beginning to confirm it. What we call "matter" is energy organized through a field of intelligence.

Your heartbeat, your nervous system, your thoughts, and your emotions do not exist in isolation from the rest of the universe. They arise within the same unified field that shapes stars, galaxies, oceans, and time itself. There is no hard boundary between you and the cosmos. Your body is a localized expression of universal intelligence.

This realization dissolves the illusion of isolation that has dominated human thinking for centuries. You are not a machine assembled from inert parts. You are a living, conscious pattern continuously held within a responsive field of life. When this understanding moves from idea to embodiment, it reorganizes how you experience existence itself.

Consciousness as the Foundation of Reality

For generations, mainstream neuroscience taught that consciousness is an accidental byproduct of the brain, a kind of biochemical side effect of neurons firing. In that view, awareness is something produced by matter.

However, research in neuroscience, quantum physics, near-death experience studies, and consciousness science is increasingly suggesting another possibility: consciousness may not arise from matter. Matter may arise within consciousness.

If this is so, awareness is not simply something you possess. It is something you participate in. Your thoughts are not sealed private events trapped inside your head. They are patterns of information moving through a wider field. Your beliefs are not only psychological habits; they are organizing principles that influence biological expression.

Your emotions are not merely chemical reactions. They are frequencies that create coherent or incoherent patterns within your internal environment. This is why chronic fear can weaken the immune system, why sustained peace can stabilize the nervous system, why prolonged stress can accelerate aging, and why experiences of meaning, love, and purpose can extend vitality beyond what biology alone might predict.

Ancient wisdom has long said, "As within, so without." Modern science now observes that perception can reshape physiology. These are two languages describing one truth.

The Universal Field and the Biology of Longevity

Longevity has often been framed as a biological lottery governed by genetics, diet, environment, and medical intervention. All of these factors matter, but they do not tell the whole story.

Epigenetics now confirms that gene expression is not fixed. Thoughts, stress levels, emotional patterns, relationships, belief systems, and environmental coherence all influence which genes become active or dormant. Your body is not a passive structure moving helplessly through time. It is a living system continually informed by consciousness.

When the internal field is coherent, cellular communication becomes efficient. When the internal field is chaotic, cellular signaling becomes distorted. The universal field is not only cosmic; it is biological. It influences how quickly your cells repair, how inflammation rises or falls, how your immune system responds, and how rapidly telomeres at the ends of chromosomes shorten.

Longevity, then, is not only a matter of prolonging time. It is a matter of staying in coherent relationship with the field that sustains life.

Why Intention Has Power

In the universal field, nothing is entirely neutral. Every thought carries information. Every emotion carries a charge. Every intention carries direction. Your body is listening continuously to your inner world. It does not simply react to external events; it responds to meaning, interpretation, expectation, and emotional tone.

When you live in chronic fear, your internal field

contracts. When you live in chronic stress, your internal field fragments. When you cultivate sustained coherence, your internal field stabilizes and strengthens. This is one of the reasons two people with the same diagnosis can have very different outcomes. Some may collapse inward under fear and hopelessness, while others may steady themselves through meaning, peace, faith, and clear intention. The difference is not only medical; it is field-based.

Intention is not wishful thinking. It is directional information introduced into a field of possibility. It invites conscious participation in what is.

The Universal Field and the Future of Medicine

Medicine is approaching one of its most significant evolutionary thresholds. It will not abandon chemistry, surgery, or pharmaceuticals; they will remain essential tools. But medicine is increasingly beginning to include frequency-based therapies, light-based treatments, bioelectromagnetic regulation, heart–brain coherence practices, sound and vibration healing, and consciousness-based interventions.

These emerging modalities do not replace traditional medicine; they complement and complete it. The body is biochemical, but it is also electromagnetic. The body is informational. The body is conscious. The most advanced medicine of the future will not be purely technological or purely spiritual; it will be integrative.

Living as a Conscious Participant in the Field

Once you begin to understand the universal field, life no longer appears as something that simply happens to you. You become a participant in reality's unfolding rather than a passive subject of circumstance.

You begin to ask different questions: What kind of internal environment are you creating? What emotional and mental frequency are you living from? Is your life expanding or contracting your energy? You also start to notice whether your nervous system feels regulated or constantly threatened, and whether your daily habits generate coherence or fragmentation.

In this way, your nervous system becomes a tuning instrument. Your breath becomes a regulator. Your awareness becomes a stabilizer. Longevity becomes a dynamic relationship with life itself, rather than a battle against time.

Breathing Exercise: Coherence Breath for Field Alignment

(Approximately three to five minutes.)

You can use this breath whenever you feel scattered, anxious, or disconnected from yourself.

Begin by sitting comfortably with both feet resting on the floor. Allow your spine to rise naturally, without strain. Place one hand on your chest and the other on your abdomen. Notice your natural breath for a few moments.

Then begin to inhale slowly through your nose for a gentle count of five. Exhale slowly through your mouth for a count of five. Continue with this smooth, even rhythm for several minutes.

As you breathe, silently repeat the words, "I am aligned. I am coherent. I am supported by life." Allow yourself to feel, even subtly, that these statements might be true. Notice your heartbeat slowing, your nervous system softening, and your body gradually returning to balance within the larger field in which you live.

Guided Meditation: Resting in the Universal Field

(Approximately eight to ten minutes.)

Find a quiet and comfortable position and gently close your eyes. Begin by noticing your breath without trying to change it. Feel air enter and leave your body in its natural rhythm.

Now imagine that with every inhale, you are drawing in a soft, luminous presence – not from somewhere far away, but from the space that already surrounds and permeates you. With every exhale, allow tension, fear, and contraction to gently release.

Begin to sense your body not only as solid matter but as a field of gentle vibration. Feel the space inside your chest. Feel the space around your body. Notice that there is no rigid line separating "you" from the space you occupy. You are within the field. The field is within you.

Rest here for several moments with no effort and no striving – only allowing.

When you feel ready, silently affirm, "I live within a universe that supports my coherence and healing." Let the words settle softly into your awareness. Then slowly bring your attention back to your breath, to the feeling of the surface beneath you, and to the sounds around you. When you are ready, gently open your eyes.

Reflection Prompts

You may wish to journal, reflect, or simply sit with questions such as these.

You might ask yourself in what ways you have been living as though you are separate from life rather than within it. You might explore which emotional or mental patterns seem to disrupt your internal sense of coherence. You can recall moments when you have felt most aligned, calm, and "in flow" with life, and consider what supported that state. You might wonder how your thoughts and intentions may be shaping your health right now. You can also ask what might change if you truly believed that the universe is intelligent and responsive to your inner world.

The universal field is not a distant abstraction. It is the living fabric in which your body, your mind, and your soul are continuously arising. Longevity depends not only on what you eat, how you move, or which treatments you receive, but on how coherently you participate in the intelligence that gives rise to all life.

In the next chapter, we move from understanding the

field to consciously living within it, exploring how awareness, energy, and intention become the daily architecture of
conscious longevity.

CHAPTER 4:
HEART–BRAIN COHERENCE: THE HIDDEN GATEWAY TO LONGEVITY, INTUITION, AND HIGHER CONSCIOUSNESS

"The heart has its reasons which reason knows nothing of."
— Blaise Pascal

Most people are taught to believe that the brain runs the body. Far fewer realize that the heart is quietly directing the brain every moment of every day. Long before modern science could measure it, ancient traditions described the heart as the center of intelligence, perception, and life force. Today, advances in neuroradiology and related fields are confirming what wisdom traditions long intuited: the heart is far more than a mechanical pump. It functions as a complex neurological, emotional, and electromagnetic center – one that profoundly influences how we think, feel, and even how we age.

The heart sends far more information to the brain than the brain sends to the heart. Its rhythmic patterns influence the autonomic nervous system, hormonal balance, immune function, and emotional regulation. The quality of this heart–brain communication helps determine whether the body stays in survival mode or shifts into restoration, growth, and repair. This dynamic relationship forms the biological foundation of heart–brain coherence – one of the most important and least understood gateways to conscious longevity.

When the Heart First Took the Lead

For most of my life, my mind led and my body followed. I learned early how to override fatigue, ignore discomfort, and push through subtle signals in the name of responsibility, productivity, and resilience. Decisions were made cognitively, often efficiently, while the body was treated as a vehicle expected to comply rather than a source of wisdom to be consulted. Over time, this quiet hierarchy – mind in command, body in service – became so normalized that I barely noticed the cost. It was only later, when energy waned and signals grew harder to dismiss, that I began to recognize how often my body had been speaking all along, patiently waiting for my attention.

I trusted my thoughts and second-guessed my feelings. I pushed through fatigue. I overrode intuition with logic. I believed that strength meant endurance and that rest was something to be earned only after everything else was done. I did not yet understand that my heart had a voice of its own.

The first time I consciously experienced the difference between thinking and coherence, I was not in a laboratory or at a retreat. I was sitting alone in a quiet room after a long, emotionally draining day. My mind raced with unfinished thoughts. My chest felt tight. My breathing had become shallow without my awareness.

I remember thinking, *I understand all of this intellectually, but something in me still feels frantic.* Instead of trying to think my way out of discomfort, I decided to do something different. I placed my hand over my heart and focused only on my breath. I inhaled slowly and exhaled even more slowly. I did not try to control my thoughts. I did not analyze my emotions. I simply breathed into the space beneath my hand.

At first, nothing seemed to change. Then, almost imperceptibly, I felt my chest soften. My breath deepened without effort. My shoulders loosened. The noise in my mind began to quiet, not because I forced it to, but because something deeper inside me had begun to lead. Within a few minutes, the urgency I had been carrying all day dissolved.

In its place, I felt something I had almost forgotten: calm clarity. I was not exhausted. I was not numb. I was not sleepy. I was present.

As I sat there, I sensed a quiet knowing that did not come from thought. It had no words, yet it felt deeply trustworthy, as if my body understood something before my mind could interpret it. That was my first conscious experience of heart–brain coherence.

At the time, I did not have scientific language for what I had just felt. I only knew that something inside me had shifted into alignment and that, in that alignment, I felt more like myself than I had in years.

Mini-Practice: A Moment of Coherent Presence

(Thirty to forty-five seconds.)

Before you read further, pause for a brief experiment.

Place one hand gently over the center of your chest. Allow your eyes to soften or close.

Take a slow, even breath in through your nose. Exhale gently through your mouth.

Repeat this one more time.

Now quietly ask within, "What am I feeling right now?" Do not search for the perfect answer. Simply notice any sensation in your chest, any subtle softening or resistance, any feeling of warmth, tightness, or ease. You have just given your heart a moment to speak and your mind a moment to listen. This is the beginning of coherence — not as a concept, but as an experience.

In the weeks that followed that first experience, I began to practice this consciously. I placed my attention on my heart, slowed my breath, and gently evoked a feeling of gratitude, calm, or appreciation. What surprised me was how quickly my body responded. My sleep improved. My reactions became less sharp. Situations that once felt overwhelming became more manageable. My intuition felt clearer – not louder or dramatic, but steadier, as though my nervous system had rediscovered its natural rhythm.

Later, when I studied the science of heart–brain coherence, everything I had felt suddenly made sense. I learned that the heart communicates with the brain through neural, hormonal, and electromagnetic pathways. I learned that when heart rhythms become coherent – smooth, ordered, and harmonious – brain waves become more organized, stress hormones decrease, and the body shifts from survival mode into regenerative mode.

What I had discovered through experience, science now confirmed. Coherence, I realized, was not something I had to earn, fix, or force. It was the natural state my system returned to once I stopped driving it with urgency and fear.

Soon afterward, another moment anchored this understanding for me. I was facing a decision that would once have filled me with anxiety. In the past, I would have made long lists of pros and cons, consulted several people, and replayed every possibility in my mind. This time, I paused. I centered my breathing. I brought my awareness gently to my heart and waited – not for an argument or a reason, but for resonance.

The answer did not arrive as a sentence in my mind. It arrived as a feeling of quiet certainty. In that instant, I realized something profound: intuition is not mysterious. It is coherence speaking.

When the heart and brain move in harmony, perception becomes clearer. When perception becomes clearer, decisions become cleaner. When the nervous system is regulated, the body ages differently. Healing accelerates. Longevity becomes less of a struggle against time and more of a partnership with it.

I had spent years trying to outthink my life. Through

coherence, I finally began to listen to it.

The more I practiced heart–brain coherence, the more I noticed subtle but powerful changes. My sense of time softened. I felt less rushed, even when my days remained full. I recovered more quickly from emotional stress. My body felt lighter – not because my life suddenly became easy, but because I was no longer carrying everything through tension alone.

Perhaps most unexpectedly, I began to trust myself in a new way. Not just the self that plans and performs, but the self that senses, feels, and quietly knows. I began to understand that coherence was not just a wellness tool. It was a gateway – a gateway into intuition, emotional regulation, higher awareness, and conscious longevity itself.

For much of my life, my heart and mind functioned as separate instruments. In coherence, they began to play in unison, and life responded with a new sense of harmony.

The Biology of Coherence

Heart–brain coherence is a measurable physiological state in which the rhythm of the heart becomes smooth, ordered, and harmonious, and the nervous system synchronizes into balance. In this state, the body functions with maximum efficiency and minimal internal friction. The brain receives clear signals of safety. Stress hormones soften. Inflammation begins to quiet. Cellular repair mechanisms activate more readily. Energy that was once diverted into defense becomes available for healing, creativity, and vitality.

In incoherence, by contrast, the heart rhythm is jagged and erratic. The nervous system stays on alert. The body behaves as though danger is present, even when life appears outwardly stable. Over time, this chronic low-grade stress accelerates biological aging. Telomeres shorten more rapidly. Immune resilience weakens. Sleep becomes shallow. Emotional regulation becomes harder. Many people live in this state of subtle incoherence for so long that they do not realize a different experience is possible.

Coherence is not the same as simple relaxation. People can relax their muscles while their inner world remains tense and guarded. Coherence is a deeper alignment in which emotional state, nervous system activity, and heart rhythm synchronize into a stable, regenerative pattern. It is not passive. It is an intelligent internal organization that allows the body to function as an integrated whole instead of as separate systems competing for balance.

From the perspective of longevity, coherence is profoundly significant. The body ages fastest under unrelenting urgency, emotional suppression, and chronic nervous system dysregulation. Coherence slows the internal experience of time. It restores natural rhythm. It signals to the body that it is safe to repair, to regenerate, and to rest. No supplement, diet, or device can fully override a nervous system that believes it is under constant threat. Coherence must come first.

Aging is often described in molecular terms, yet beneath every molecular process lies an emotional and neurological influence. Chronic fear constricts the vascular system and burdens the heart; unresolved grief can suppress immune function; persistent resentment elevates inflammatory markers; and prolonged loneliness is increasingly associated with accelerated cognitive decline. Conversely, emotional states such as gratitude, compassion, forgiveness, and love tend to stabilize heart rhythm and strengthen vagal tone, which directly supports immune resilience and nervous system regulation.

These emotional states are not merely noble sentiments. They are measurable biological forces that shape how the body ages across decades. Heart–brain coherence is the mechanism through which emotional life becomes physiological reality. The way we feel becomes what the body expresses. For this reason, coherence is not a spiritual luxury. It is a central practice of conscious longevity.

The Inner Triad of Consciousness Evolution: Coherence, Intuition, and Higher Consciousness

One of the most fascinating aspects of coherence is its relationship to intuition. In coherent states, the brain becomes more flexible and integrative. Mental noise softens. Pattern recognition sharpens. Many people notice clearer insight, deeper discernment, and a quiet sense of inner knowing when they are coherent. This is not supernatural. It is neurological. When stress hormones decrease and the limbic system relaxes, the brain regains access to broader perception. Intuition becomes coherent perception.

Higher consciousness also emerges more naturally in coherent states. Expanded awareness does not require escaping the body. It requires alignment within the body. Heart–brain coherence stabilizes the internal environment so that awareness can widen without being continuously pulled back into survival patterns. The body becomes a hospitable vessel for consciousness rather than a battleground of tension and defense. For this reason, spiritual traditions across time have emphasized the heart as a center of awakening – not only symbolically but functionally.

Modern life, however, unintentionally conditions incoherence. Constant stimulation, digital overload, emotional suppression, relentless pace, and fragmented rest continually strain the nervous system. Over time, low-grade stress becomes so familiar that regulation feels foreign. Stillness may register as unsafe. Quiet may feel empty. Rest may be dismissed as unproductive. In this normalization of incoherence, accelerated aging often follows – quietly and unseen.

Conscious longevity restores coherence as a daily biological practice. The body learns through repeated shifts in state, not through intellectual insight alone. Even a few minutes of coherence practice each day can improve heart rate variability, stabilize mood, strengthen immune regulation, deepen sleep, and increase emotional resilience. Over time, coherence becomes not an occasional technique but the internal climate from which one lives.

This is where conscious longevity becomes embodied rather than theoretical. The body is no longer forced toward health through discipline alone. It is invited into health through regulation, rhythm, and presence.

The Three Relationships That Shape Your Longevity

Longevity is often described as a biological pursuit – an effort to preserve the body, maintain vitality, and extend the number of years lived. But conscious longevity is something far more holistic and profound. It is not merely about living longer. It is about living with presence, coherence, and alignment. It is about inhabiting your life rather than rushing through it. And at the core of this approach lie three foundational relationships: the relationship with the body, the relationship with the mind, and the relationship with meaning.

Each of these relationships influences the others, forming an interconnected system. When one is neglected, the whole system is affected; when one is nourished, the entire field of life begins to shift. Conscious longevity is not an abstract concept but an ongoing conversation among these three relationships – unfolding moment by moment, breath by breath, and choice by choice.

1. The Relationship With the Body: Listening Instead of Controlling

For much of my life, I treated my body as a vehicle that needed to perform. I pushed through fatigue. I dismissed discomfort. I interpreted symptoms as inconveniences rather than as communication. Over time, this created a quiet war between what my mind demanded and what my body needed.

It was only when I began listening to my body – truly listening – that longevity revealed its deeper architecture. I discovered that the body does not speak in language. It speaks in sensation. In tightness or ease, in warmth or constriction, in intuition that rises from places deeper than thought.

In conscious longevity, the body becomes a partner, not a project. It becomes a teacher with its own intelligence. To listen to it is to strengthen vitality. To ignore it is to weaken the foundation of your entire life.

2. The Relationship With the Mind: From Noise to Navigation

The mind is a magnificent instrument – creative, analytical, persistent, and capable of extraordinary insight. But the mind is also conditioned. It repeats patterns inherited from childhood, from society, from fear, from survival. Left unchecked, it can drown out intuition and overwhelm the body's natural rhythms.

Conscious longevity does not ask you to silence the mind, but to become aware of its patterns. Your thoughts shape your chemistry. Your perceptions shape your biology. What you anticipate, fear, imagine, and repeat becomes part of the internal environment in which your cells operate.

The mind becomes a tool for longevity only when you recognize that you are not your thoughts – you are the awareness observing them.

3. The Relationship With Meaning: What Gives Your Life Its Coherence

The body cannot thrive for long without meaning. Meaning is the emotional and spiritual framework that gives direction to your days and organizes your nervous system around hope, purpose, and coherence.

Meaning does not need to be grand, a mission, or a legacy. Meaning can be rooted in relationships, creativity, faith, service, beauty, or the simple desire to grow consciously throughout your lifetime. Without meaning, longevity becomes effortful and hollow. With meaning, longevity becomes natural – an extension of the desire to remain awake to life.

Meaning stabilizes your biology. It softens fear. It regulates the nervous system. It anchors you in a state where healing and expansion remain possible.

The Moment These Three Relationships Came Together

There was a morning when I realized these three relationships were no longer separate in my life. I was making breakfast, feeling the warmth of the pan in my hand, listening to my breath as I moved, and reflecting on what I hoped the day would bring.

My body felt grounded. My mind felt spacious. My heart felt connected to something larger than the tasks ahead.

In that ordinary moment, I understood that conscious longevity was not something I practiced occasionally – it was becoming the way I lived. These three relationships had become the quiet compass guiding every choice I made.

And this is what I want for you – not perfection, not control, not a demanding wellness routine, but a daily blueprint that supports coherence in simple, accessible ways.

Breathing Exercise: Coherent Heart Breathing

(Approximately five minutes.)

You may wish to try the following practice to experience heart–brain coherence more directly.

Sit comfortably with your spine upright and place one hand gently over the center of your chest. Allow your eyes to soften or close. Begin by noticing your natural breath for a few moments without trying to change it.

Then, slowly inhale through your nose to a gentle count of five. Exhale through your mouth to the same count of five. Imagine that the breath is moving in and out through the area beneath your hand, as if your heart itself is breathing. Continue with this smooth, even rhythm.

As you breathe, invite a gentle emotional quality to arise – perhaps gratitude, compassion, or a sense of safety. There is no need to force a strong emotion. Simply allow a memory, image, or feeling tone to soften your body as you continue breathing through the heart area.

Remain with this slow, even heart-focused breathing for several minutes. When you feel complete, pause before returning to your natural breath. Notice any shift in your body, your mind, or your emotional state. You have just practiced heart–brain coherence.

Guided Meditation: Entering the Coherent Field

(Approximately eight to ten minutes.)

Find a quiet place where you can sit or lie down comfortably. Gently close your eyes and bring your attention to the area around your heart. Feel the subtle rise and fall of your breath. With each inhale, imagine the space around your heart becoming warmer, steadier, and more spacious. With each exhale, allow any internal pressure to release.

Begin to visualize your heart rhythm as smooth and even, like gentle waves moving across calm water. Imagine your brain responding to this signal from the heart, softening and organizing in response. Allow your entire nervous system to receive the message that it is safe to rest and restore.

Silently affirm to yourself, "It is safe for my body to heal and regulate." Let the words land gently inside you. Stay with the feeling of safety and steadiness for several breaths.

When you feel ready, ask quietly within, "What becomes possible for me when I live from coherence?" Do not force an answer. It may arrive as a feeling, an image, a phrase, or simply a sense of spaciousness. Trust that the question itself plants a seed in your awareness.

Remain in this coherent field for a few more breaths. Then begin to deepen your breathing slightly. Become aware of the surface beneath you, the sounds around you, and the weight of your body. When you are ready, gently open your eyes. You have just experienced what it is like to enter a coherent inner state.

Reflection Prompts

You may wish to journal about your experience or reflect on the following questions:

- When in my life do I feel most coherent and regulated, and what conditions seem to support that state?

- What daily habits or patterns quietly generate incoherence for me, even if I have normalized them?

- How does my body signal the difference between being regulated and being stressed?

- In what ways might emotional safety – or the lack of it – be influencing my aging process?

- What shifts when I allow my heart to lead, rather than following only the urgency of my mind?

Heart–brain coherence reveals that longevity is not created through effort alone, but through rhythm, regulation, and a compassionate relationship with the nervous system. In the next chapter, we move from understanding to embodiment as we explore the daily practices that stabilize coherence, support awareness, and quietly reshape the internal environment in which longevity unfolds. Chapter 4 becomes the living blueprint for conscious longevity in everyday life.

CHAPTER 5:
THE QUANTUM FIELD OF HEALING: HOW ENERGY, INTENTION, AND CONSCIOUSNESS SHAPE THE BODY

"The greatest discovery of my generation is that human beings can alter their lives by altering their attitudes of mind."
— William James

At the deepest level of existence, the body is not simply a structure of tissues and organs. It is a vibrating field of information, continuously shaped by awareness, emotion, and meaning. What appears solid is, in truth, a dynamic pattern of energy responding to the invisible field in which it lives. This is the quantum field of healing – the subtle architecture through which consciousness and biology are forever intertwined.

A Short Story of Realization

My understanding of this field did not arrive with drama or revelation. It came quietly, during an evening when I was simply exhausted. I sat alone, eyes closed, breathing slowly and without effort. My mind softened. My body warmed. And in that softened state, I felt something unexpected. My body no longer seemed dense and heavy. It felt spacious, porous, almost luminous, as though I were made of gentle waves rather than solid matter.

In that moment, I sensed something unmistakable: my body was not waiting for an external force to fix it. It was waiting for me to stop constricting it with fear, tension, and habit. It was waiting for coherence. The realization did not come through thought. It came through sensation, through a subtle knowing that my cells were listening to me, responding to the quality of my attention. From that evening forward, I understood that healing was not separate from my consciousness. Healing was shaped by it.

Mini Practice: Entering the Field of Cellular Harmony

Settle into a comfortable position, allowing your spine to rise naturally as if it were being lifted gently from above. Place one hand over your heart and the other over your lower abdomen. Feel the warmth of your palms as they make contact with your body and let that warmth remind you that you are safe, held, and supported.

Take a slow inhale through your nose, letting the breath move down into the lower hand. As you inhale, imagine that you are drawing in coherence – a soft, steady light that knows where to go within your body. As you exhale through your mouth, imagine that your breath carries out any resistance, tension, or internal noise that no longer serves your system. Allow your exhale to feel longer than your inhale, as if you are giving your body ample space to release.

On the next breath, bring gentle awareness to one place in your body that feels tight, tender, fatigued, or simply in need of attention today. Do not try to change it. Do not judge it. Simply acknowledge it the way you would acknowledge a child who has approached you with a story to tell. Consider that this area is not a problem to fix but a message to receive.

As you breathe, imagine that the coherent light flowing in through your lungs moves effortlessly toward this area, not to force healing but to offer presence. Allow that light to wrap softly around the sensation, as though you were placing a warm blanket over something cold and shivering.

Inwardly whisper to that part of your body, "You are not alone. I am with you."

Then whisper, "You are already within the field of healing."

Feel the subtle shift that occurs when the body is met with compassion instead of pressure. Notice how even the smallest acknowledgment begins to reorganize the internal field. Let your breath continue to guide you. With each inhale, feel the light of coherence expand. With each exhale, feel your body soften further into receptivity.

Stay here for a few more breaths, not searching for results, simply resting in relationship with your own energy. When you feel ready, release your hands gently to your lap. Offer your body a final quiet affirmation: "We heal together."

Carry this sensation of partnership with you as you return to your day. Healing is not a distant possibility. It is a living process already unfolding inside you, breath by breath.

What This Entire Book Has Been Leading Toward

Every chapter of this book has been preparing the ground for this final truth. Conscious longevity is not built on lifestyle alone, nor on medical intervention, nor on spiritual practice in isolation. It emerges from the way consciousness interacts with biology – how presence softens the nervous system, how meaning organizes physiology, how awareness stabilizes the internal environment in which cells operate.

To understand healing at this deeper level is to understand that you are not a passive recipient of your physiology. You are a participant in the field that shapes it. When your inner world becomes coherent, your biology shifts. When your intention becomes steady, your cells orient around it.

When your emotions shift into states such as gratitude or compassion, your body receives signals that restoration is possible.

Coherence as the Body's Healing State

Coherence is the state in which the nervous system relaxes into safety, the heart settles into a harmonious rhythm, and the body returns to its natural capacity for repair. This state is not simply calmness; it is alignment – mind, heart, and body moving in the same direction. When coherence is present, stress hormones recede, inflammation quiets, and regeneration becomes efficient. The body is built to heal in coherence. It struggles to heal in fragmentation.

Intention as the Direction of Energy

Intention, when grounded in safety rather than force, becomes a quiet directive within the quantum field. It is not wishful thinking; it is a subtle organizing principle that shapes the informational environment in which cells operate. Modern research demonstrates that expectation and belief alter physiology. The placebo effect reveals this truth with extraordinary clarity: the body responds not to the sugar pill but to the meaning assigned to it. Intention becomes biologically believable only when the nervous system feels safe enough to receive it.

Elevated Emotion as the Fuel of Transformation

Emotions such as gratitude, love, and compassion are not sentimental experiences. They are biological regulators that change the electromagnetic field of the heart, increase immune strength, and deepen neural plasticity. Elevated emotion signals to the body that life is safe, that opening is possible, and that repair can begin. Healing cannot unfold in fear; it requires an atmosphere in which the body feels held rather than threatened.

And now, and always, that healing is not something distant you must chase. It is something that unfolds when you live in gentle partnership with the field of life moving through you.

You have traveled far to arrive here, to this deeper understanding of who you are and how your body listens. You are not separate from the intelligence that heals you; you never were. And now you know how to enter it – breath by breath, moment by moment, with awareness, compassion, and trust.

Breathing Exercise: Entering the Quantum Field of Coherence

(Approximately five minutes.)

- Sit comfortably with your spine upright and your shoulders relaxed.
- Inhale slowly through your nose for a count of six.
- Exhale slowly through your mouth for a count of eight.
- With each inhale, silently repeat, "I receive coherence."
- With each exhale, silently repeat, "I release resistance."

Allow your breath to become smooth and spacious, as if you are breathing not only into your lungs but into your entire field of being. Continue for several minutes. When finished, return to natural breathing and notice the subtle quality of your internal state.

Guided Meditation: Healing Within the Quantum Field

(Approximately eight to ten minutes.)

Close your eyes gently and bring awareness to your breathing. Feel the natural rise and fall of your chest and abdomen.

Now imagine your entire body as a field of light and

information rather than solid matter. Sense this field as soft, responsive, and intelligent.

Bring gentle attention to any area of your body that feels tense, fatigued, or in need of healing. Without forcing change, simply place awareness there and silently affirm, **"You are already within the field of restoration."**

Allow this awareness to remain for several breaths.

Now imagine coherence gently rippling through your entire body like a wave of quiet order, harmonizing every cell, every system, every layer. Rest in this sensation for several minutes.

When you are ready, bring your attention back to the support beneath you, the sounds around you, and slowly open your eyes.

Reflection Prompts

If you would like to integrate this chapter more deeply, you might reflect or journal on questions like these:

1. How does viewing my body as an intelligent energy field change the way I relate to healing?
2. Where in my life do I experience the most coherence – and where do I feel the most fragmentation?
3. How might my emotional states be shaping my physical health right now?
4. What would it mean for me to heal in partnership with consciousness rather than in opposition to my body?
5. What one simple daily practice could I commit to that supports coherence at the deepest level – breath, gratitude, stillness, honest emotion, or something else?
6. You have traveled through the awakening of consciousness, the multidimensional nature of the soul, the architecture of awareness, the future of

humanity, and finally into the quantum field where all healing ultimately unfolds.

What remains now is not more information – but embodiment.

Conscious longevity is not achieved by understanding alone. It is revealed through how you breathe, how you listen, how you rest, how you relate, how you make meaning of time, and how you participate in the field of life each day.

You do not need to master the universe. You need only to live in coherent relationship with it. And in that relationship, healing continues. Longevity unfolds. Awakening deepens. The soul remembers. And life – infinitely intelligent – responds.

CHAPTER 6:
HEALING ACROSS DIMENSIONS: HOW ENERGY, EMOTION, AND CONSCIOUSNESS SHAPE THE BODY AND EXTEND HUMAN LIFE

"The wound is the place where the Light enters you."
— Rumi

Healing is not only the repair of the body. It is the restoration of coherence – between your biology, your emotions, your energy, your relationships, and the meaning you make of your life. For centuries, medicine focused almost exclusively on the physical dimension, treating the body as an isolated structure that breaks and must be repaired. But the human being is not an isolated structure. We are interwoven dimensions of memory, perception, and intelligence, each dimension shaping the others in powerful ways.

When I Realized My Healing Was Bigger Than My Body

For much of my life, I believed what many of us are taught: if something hurts, you treat the body; if something is wrong, you look for a physical cause. Doctors were my first and last stop. Tests guided my understanding. Recommendations shaped my decisions. And for a long time, this was enough.

But slowly, I began noticing something subtle and unsettling. Some symptoms returned even when the tests were normal. Exhaustion lingered despite rest. Discomfort shifted unpredictably, loosening one week only to tighten the next, without any clear physical reason.

I told myself these fluctuations were part of aging. But something inside me remained unconvinced.

The turning point came during a season of deliberate inner care. I was slowing down, practicing breathwork, nourishing myself with intention, and paying closer attention to my internal world. Yet during this time – when I felt more conscious than ever before – an unexpected physical challenge appeared.

It was not dramatic, but it was persistent. A discomfort that refused to be ignored. I always had appointments, tests, instructions. I did everything right. Yet something didn't add up.

My symptoms did not respond only to treatment. They responded to my emotional state.

On days when I felt calm and connected, my body softened. On days marked by overwhelm or quiet distress, the discomfort sharpened. At first, I resisted the idea that emotion could matter this much. But the pattern was unmistakable.

One evening, after weeks of observing this strange rhythm, I sat alone for a long time. A realization rose within me with gentle certainty: **My body was not simply responding to medicine. It was responding to my inner life.**

That single insight changed everything. Instead of looking only at the physical sensation, I asked myself: *What emotion have I not expressed? What fear have I not acknowledged? What tension have I learned to live with?*

The answers were not always comfortable. I saw how I frequently put others' needs ahead of my own. I saw how often I swallowed truth to avoid conflict. I saw how much quiet tension my body had been carrying for years.

But as soon as I began listening – truly listening – subtle shifts emerged. My chest loosened when I spoke honestly. My energy lifted when I set boundaries without guilt. My breath deepened when I allowed myself to grieve old losses instead of minimizing them. And gradually, almost imperceptibly at first, my physical symptoms began to change.

I had not changed my diagnosis. I had changed my relationship with myself. My body was not failing me. My body was speaking to me. And when I listened, it responded.

As the weeks passed, I felt changes that medicine alone could not explain: a softening of old tightness, a release of unspoken emotional weight, a new fullness in my breath. My body felt less like an object and more like an intelligent partner – always communicating, always adapting to the climate of my inner world.

Healing, I realized, was not something happening *to* me. It was something happening *through* me.

Healing Is Multidimensional

To understand conscious longevity, you must expand your understanding of healing itself. The body does not respond only to chemistry. It responds to the emotional weather inside you, the relational field that surrounds you, the meaning you assign to your experiences, and the energetic coherence moving through your system.

The physical dimension is the most visible – but it is not the beginning. Beneath the body lies the nervous system. Beneath the nervous system lies emotional patterns.

Beneath emotional patterns lie perception and meaning. Beneath meaning lies energy – your most subtle, responsive layer. And beneath energy lies consciousness itself.

The body is the final expression of all these layers interacting continuously.

This does not mean illness is "your fault." It means insight is possible.

The nervous system is especially central. It is the

translator between experience and biology. When the system perceives threat, healing slows. When it perceives safety, healing accelerates. The body heals not through force, but through regulation, coherence, and awareness.

And this coherence is influenced by every dimension of your life.

Healing Across Dimensions in Practice

Healing across dimensions is not theoretical. It is lived. It is sensed. And it can be cultivated daily.

Below are simple, accessible practices – one for each dimension – to help you enter coherence from wherever you stand.

A Five-Dimensional Reset

1. Physical Dimension – Softening the Breath

Take one slow inhale through the nose. Exhale twice as long through the mouth.

Repeat three times. This signals safety to your nervous system and invites your body out of contraction.

2. Emotional Dimension – Naming Gently

Place your hand over your heart and whisper the name of the emotion you feel: *sadness, fear, uncertainty, anger, overwhelm.*

Naming an emotion reduces its intensity and frees trapped energy.

3. Energetic Dimension – Clearing the Field

Close your eyes. Imagine a warm light at the crown of your head gently cascading down your body like a waterfall.

Let it wash through you, clearing tension as it moves.

This restores flow and interrupts stress-based stagnation.

4. Relational Dimension – One True Connection

Think of one person you feel safe with.

Imagine sending them a silent blessing, *May you be well. May you feel supported.*

This shifts your nervous system into connection rather than isolation.

5. Meaning Dimension – Reframing the Moment

Ask yourself: *What might this experience be asking me to see or learn?*

Not as punishment, but as invitation. Meaning transforms stress into insight.

Mini-Practice: Listening to Symptom as Messenger

If you wish, pause for a moment now. Bring to mind one area of your body that feels uncomfortable, tense, or weary. Gently place a hand over or near that area if possible. Take a slow breath through your nose and a long, soft breath out through your mouth. Then quietly ask, "If this symptom were a messenger rather than an enemy, what might it be trying to tell me?"

You do not need a clear answer. Simply making space for the question is a form of healing across dimensions, because you are allowing the body, emotion, and awareness to enter into relationship.

Healing as Reorganization of Coherence

Conscious longevity asks us to expand our understanding of healing. Every symptom carries more than chemistry. It carries history. It carries stress. It carries adaptation. It carries the stories the nervous system has learned to tell about life and safety. The body is not only responding to the present moment. It responds to the cumulative emotional and energetic climate it has lived through.

This does not mean that illness is created by thought alone or that suffering is the sign of insufficient positivity. It means that the human system is inherently multidimensional. Biology, emotion, and consciousness are inseparable expressions of one continuous field of experience. Healing that ignores this complexity often treats effects while deeper causes remain unresolved.

Viewed across dimensions, healing becomes not only the correction of dysfunction, but the reorganization of coherence. The physical dimension of the body is the most visible. It is where pain is felt, where disease is diagnosed, where interventions are applied. Yet the physical body is shaped from upstream forces that cannot be seen on imaging or blood tests alone.

Beneath tissue lies the nervous system. Beneath the nervous system lies emotional patterning. Beneath emotional patterning lies perception, meaning, and belief. Beneath awareness lies subtle energy, the medium through which all these layers communicate. The body is a downstream expression of all these dimensions interacting continuously.

When emotional stress becomes chronic, it reorganizes posture, breathing, digestion, and circulation. When unresolved grief lingers, it alters immune function and hormonal balance. When long-held fear becomes a background frequency, it shapes vascular tone, sleep depth, and inflammatory load. These shifts do not occur because the body is malfunctioning. They occur because the body is adapting to conditions it must repeatedly endure.

From a survival perspective, these adaptations are intelligent. The problem is not that the body adapts; the problem arises when it must adapt to conditions that never resolve. Healing across dimensions begins when unresolved internal states are allowed to reorganize rather than simply endured.

Emotion is one of the most powerful architects of the body. Emotion is not abstract. It is neurochemical movement traveling through tissue, blood, nerves, and breath. Every emotional state corresponds to a physiological pattern. Fear constricts. Grief collapses. Anger mobilizes. Joy expands. Safety opens.

When emotion moves freely, the body remains

adaptable. When emotion is chronically suppressed, the body must carry that unresolved energy somewhere else. Over time, suppression becomes structure. What began as a temporary response becomes a long-term posture.

Healing across dimensions does not require endlessly revisiting the past. It asks that what has been held be allowed to move, integrate, and complete its cycle of expression within the safety of present awareness.

The nervous system plays a central role as translator between experience and biology. It decides moment by moment whether the body should orient toward defense or toward restoration. When the nervous system remains locked in a perception of threat, healing resources remain limited. When the nervous system senses safety, the body shifts spontaneously into repair.

True healing does not begin with force. It begins with safety.

Safety is not merely the absence of obvious danger. It is the felt sense that life is navigable, that experience can be tolerated, that the present moment does not overwhelm the system. For many people, the most profound barrier to healing is not the severity of symptoms, but the absence of sustained safety in the nervous system.

Consciousness enters the healing process as the great integrator. It allows awareness to move into sensation without being consumed by it. It allows memory to surface without overwhelming the present. It allows pain to be felt without becoming identity. It allows fear to pass through the body without becoming permanent residence.

Healing across dimensions requires consciousness because awareness prevents experience from becoming trapped. Energy is the medium through which this integration takes place. Wherever attention goes, energy follows. Wherever energy remains restricted, healing stagnates. Wherever energy is allowed to circulate with awareness and safety, healing accelerates.

From this perspective, symptoms are not enemies to be

silenced. They are messages traveling across dimensions, re-flecting how the system is organizing in response to both past and present. Healing becomes the process of listening deeply enough for those messages to complete their function.

Many people fear listening to the body because they imagine that what they hear will overwhelm them. Yet the body has been waiting to be heard. It carries memory not to punish, but to protect. When awareness enters with gentleness rather than force, the body often loosens its grip on old stories far more readily than we expect.

Healing across dimensions also involves the relationship between identity and physiology. How you see yourself shapes how your body responds to stress. When you see yourself as fragile, the body tightens. When you see yourself as resilient, the body opens. When identity becomes fused with illness, the nervous system adapts to sustain that identity. When identity gradually shifts toward healing, the nervous system reorganizes toward restoration.

This is not a denial of suffering; it is a recognition that meaning shapes matter. One of the quiet shifts of conscious longevity is moving from the question, "How do I fix the body?" to also asking, "How is my body responding to the way I relate to life?"

Healing across dimensions becomes possible when you stop living against the body and begin living with it. This does not mean abandoning medical intervention. It means widening the field within which medicine operates. Physical treatments work most effectively when the internal environment is coherent – when the nervous system feels safe, when emotions are allowed to move, when awareness is present and compassionate.

Longevity, from this integrated perspective, is not extended merely by suppressing symptoms. It is extended by restoring flow across dimensions so that the system can renew itself with less internal resistance. Human beings heal not only through chemistry, but through relationship – with themselves, with others, with meaning, and with life itself.

This is why isolation often accelerates suffering, while connection often accelerates repair. The nervous system is inherently relational. It evolved to regulate in the presence of others. Touch, voice, eye contact, and shared emotional experience all profoundly influence healing responses. Conscious longevity cannot truly be cultivated in isolation from meaningful relationship.

What differentiates healing across dimensions from purely conventional approaches is not a rejection of science, but an expansion of the field in which science is applied. It recognizes that the body does not heal in pieces. It heals as a whole.

In this view, the future of medicine is neither purely physical nor purely energetic, neither strictly clinical nor purely contemplative. At its core, it is integrative – honoring structure and story, chemistry and consciousness, body and time.

As this understanding deepens, aging itself begins to transform. Instead of appearing as a one-directional march toward decline, aging becomes a continual opportunity for integration. Each decade carries not only loss, but the possibility of reorganizing unresolved layers of experience into greater coherence.

Extended life is not merely the prolongation of survival. It is the widening of the field in which healing can continue to unfold. When healing is allowed to move across dimensions, it often reaches places the mind alone could never touch.

Breathing Exercise: Restoring Dimensional Flow

(Approximately five minutes.)

You may wish to try the following breath practice to support healing across the layers of your experience.

Sit comfortably with your spine upright and place one hand on your heart and the other on your abdomen. Begin by noticing your natural breath and the gentle movement beneath your hands. Then inhale slowly through your nose for a count of five, allowing both your chest and abdomen to expand. Exhale slowly through your mouth for a count of seven, allowing both areas to soften completely.

As you exhale, silently repeat the phrase, "I release what no longer needs to be held." As you inhale, silently repeat, "I welcome integration." Continue this pattern for several minutes. When you feel complete, allow your breath to return to its natural rhythm and notice any subtle shift in sensation, emotion, or clarity.

Guided Meditation: Integrating Across Dimensions

(Approximately eight to ten minutes.)

Find a quiet place and gently close your eyes. Bring your awareness first to the physical sensations of your body. Notice areas of tension, ease, warmth, coolness, or neutrality. There is nothing to change. You are simply meeting your body as it is.

Next, bring awareness to your emotional state. Without needing to name it, sense the general tone of your inner world – perhaps restlessness, calm, sadness, curiosity, or something more subtle. Allow whatever is present to be there, without pushing it away and without clinging to it.

Now gently bring awareness to the quiet field beneath both sensation and emotion, the space of consciousness that is aware of all of this. Imagine these three layers – body, emotion, and awareness – softly aligning within you, like overlapping circles of gentle light.

With each breath, feel these layers communicating more freely. You might sense that the body is sharing information with emotion, emotion is sharing information with awareness, and awareness is holding everything in kindness. Silently affirm, "My system is learning to heal as one."

Rest in this integrated state for several breaths, allowing your body, your heart, and your consciousness to share the same space. When you are ready, bring your attention back to the room, notice the surface beneath you, and open your eyes.

Reflection Prompts

If you would like to deepen this chapter's insights, you may wish to reflect or journal in response to a few gentle questions.

You might explore how you currently relate to your healing process. Consider whether you have been trying to heal only at the physical level while ignoring emotional, energetic, or relational dimensions of your experience. You may notice which emotions feel most closely linked to your physical sensations right now and how your sense of safety – or lack of it – affects your vitality. You might ask how meaningful relationships, or the absence of them, influence your healing. Finally, you can contemplate what healing would mean for you beyond the simple absence of symptoms – perhaps as a sense of wholeness, coherence, or trust.

As healing expands across dimensions, awareness naturally begins to question the nature of consciousness itself. If the body responds to emotion, memory, and meaning, what is the deeper field through which awareness travels?

In the next chapter, we move into the multidimensional nature of the soul – exploring how awareness may extend beyond a single lifetime, how experience may travel across layers of being, and what this expanded view of existence can mean for conscious longevity.

CHAPTER 7:
CONSCIOUS LONGEVITY:
EXTENDING LIFE THROUGH
AWARENESS, ENERGY, AND
INTENTION

*"The quality of your life is determined by the quality
of your awareness."*
— Eckhart Tolle

Longevity is not created by time alone. It is created by
your relationship with awareness, with energy, and with intention. Time may carry the body forward, but it is awareness that determines how that time is experienced, how the
body adapts, and how vitality is either preserved or quietly
depleted along the way.

For centuries, human beings viewed aging as something
that simply happened to them – a largely uncontrollable biological process shaped by inheritance and chance. Today,
science tells a more complex and far more hopeful story.
Aging is not merely passive; it is a dynamic, responsive conversation between your inner life and your biology.

When Longevity Became a Living Choice

For a long time, I thought of longevity as something external – something shaped by genetics, doctors,

medications, and luck. I believed you either aged well or you did not. I believed time was the ultimate authority over the body. Without ever deliberately choosing it, I accepted the idea that decline was inevitable.

That belief was gently but unmistakably interrupted during a season when I was paying closer attention than ever before – not only to my thoughts but to my energy. I began to notice how differently I felt at different times of the day, how certain conversations left me drained while others lifted me, and how some choices nourished me while others, just as quietly, depleted me.

For the first time, I recognized that energy was not an abstraction. It was the invisible atmosphere I lived in every moment.

One afternoon became a clear turning point. I had just come from a medical appointment. All my numbers were "normal." I was told, kindly and efficiently, that I was doing "fine for my age." Those words followed me home. *Fine for my age.* They landed in my body like a small, heavy stone.

That evening, I sat alone in my living room with the lights dimmed and the house silent. I placed one hand on my chest and one on my abdomen and simply breathed. As my breath settled, a clear thought arose – not from fear, but from a deeply honest place: *I do not want to live fine for my age. I want to live fully alive in my body at every age.*

That was the moment longevity stopped being an abstract concept and became personal. I realized I was no longer willing to outsource my relationship with time to statistics and averages. I wanted to participate – consciously and intentionally – in shaping my vitality. From that night forward, the way I inhabited my body began to change.

I stopped thinking of my body as something quietly wearing out. I began to see it as a responsive living field of energy, constantly influenced by how I breathed, how I thought, how I felt, how I rested, how I loved, and how I made meaning of my days. I noticed how my energy shifted when I rushed instead of moving with intention. I noticed how my body responded when I spoke to myself with kindness instead of criticism. I noticed how fatigue softened when I allowed myself genuine rest rather than collapsing only when I had no strength left.

Awareness alone began to change my biology. But awareness was only the first doorway. The next shift came when I began to work consciously with intention.

I had always set goals and been productive, but I discovered that intention was not the same thing as ambition. Intention carried feeling, direction, and presence. It was not about forcing outcomes. It was about orienting my energy toward life instead of away from it.

Each morning, rather than beginning with a list of tasks, I started with a simple inner question: *How do I want to feel in my body today?* Sometimes the answer was steady. Sometimes it was open. Sometimes it was rested. Sometimes it was strong. That single question changed the tone of my entire day. I noticed that when I held a clear intention for my state of being, my nervous system seemed to reorganize around it. My breathing adjusted. My posture softened. My mind became less scattered. My body cooperated instead of resisting.

I was no longer driving myself forward. I was guiding myself forward. And something extraordinary began to happen: my experience of time started to change. Days no longer felt like something to endure. They became spaces to inhabit. My energy at the end of the day did not feel completely spent. I was not necessarily doing less, but I was losing less energy through tension, worry, and self-abandonment.

I began to understand that the greatest thief of longevity is not age itself, but unconscious depletion – the gradual draining of energy, resilience, and coherence that occurs when stress goes unrecognized and recovery is postponed. This kind of depletion builds quietly through chronic over-extension, emotional suppression, and living in a constant state of urgency. Over time, the body adapts to this strain by conserving resources, lowering vitality, and prioritizing survival over repair.

Age marks the passage of time; unconscious depletion accelerates its effects. When attention, rest, and emotional regulation are restored, the body often responds with renewed stability and capacity. In this way, longevity is shaped less by the number of years lived and more by how consciously those years are inhabited.

One morning, as I walked slowly outside just after sunrise, this understanding settled into me in a way I could feel. The air was cool. The world was quiet. My steps were unhurried. My breath was deep without effort. Suddenly, a simple truth became unmistakable: *My body is not trying to run out of time. It is always trying to return to balance.*

That insight reshaped how I related to every ache, every moment of fatigue, and every sign of aging. Rather than reading them as evidence of decline, I came to see them as invitations – to restore balance, return to coherence, replenish energy, and realign intention with how I was actually living.

I no longer asked, "How old am I?" I began asking, "How aligned am I right now?" The answers were not always comfortable, but they were always honest. There were days when I realized I had overextended myself emotionally, days when I had ignored my need for rest, and days when I had tolerated levels of stress I no longer wished to carry. Instead of criticizing myself, I made small, deliberate adjustments. I rested. I breathed. I slowed down. I chose differently.

Over time, my body began to change in ways I had not expected. I recovered more quickly from illness. I felt steadier under stress. My sleep became deeper. My clarity sharpened. My joy grew less dependent on circumstances. I was not becoming younger; I was becoming more alive.

The greatest revelation of conscious longevity for me was this: extending life is not only about adding years. It is about adding presence, coherence, and vitality to the years that are already here.

I stopped waiting for "later" to feel fully alive. I stopped assuming energy would inevitably fade into emptiness. I stopped relating to vitality as a resource that would only diminish. Instead, I began to treat energy as something that could be cultivated, protected, and renewed.

In doing so, something inside me softened for the first time in many years: the quiet fear of growing old. Aging no longer felt like an enemy approaching in the distance. It felt like a process of refinement. Longevity no longer felt like a distant medical hope. It felt like a daily, conscious relationship with life itself.

That was when I knew, without doubt, that conscious longevity was not a theory. It was a way of living I had already begun to embody.

Mini-Practice: Asking the Body, Not the Calendar

You might pause for a brief moment now and try a simple inquiry.

Allow your body to settle wherever you are. Take a slow breath in through your nose and a gentle breath out through your mouth. Then quietly ask yourself, "If I stop asking how old I am and instead ask how aligned I am, what do I notice right now?"

Let the answer arrive as sensation, emotion, or a quiet knowing. There is nothing to fix. This is simply a moment of honest contact with yourself, the kind of contact that conscious longevity is built upon.

Awareness, Energy, and Intention as Living Forces

Awareness is what allows you to enter the conversation with your body consciously. The moment you notice your breath changing under stress, you are already influencing your nervous system. The moment you recognize emotional contraction in your chest or abdomen, you begin to alter circulation, hormone release, and muscular tension. The moment you see how your pace affects your sleep and energy, you step out of automatism and into participation.

Conscious longevity does not begin with changing the body. It begins with changing your relationship to the body. Awareness does not wage war on the body; it listens. And what is truly listened to begins to soften, reorganize, and restore.

Most people live inside patterns they did not consciously choose. They breathe shallowly, carry tension without noticing, and move through days with a level of urgency that feels "normal" only because it is familiar. The nervous system adapts to these conditions and quietly adopts them as a baseline. Over time, that baseline helps shape the trajectory of aging.

Awareness disrupts unexamined conditioning. It allows you to sense when your energy is contracting and when it is expanding, to feel when something is life-giving and when it is life-draining, and to notice the precise moment just before reactivity crystallizes into physiology.

Awareness is the doorway through which every other longevity intervention must pass.

Energy is the currency through which awareness shapes the body. Every biological function depends on energy: cellular repair, immune response, neural signaling, and metabolic regulation all require the free movement of energy through tissues and systems. When energy flows freely, the body organizes itself toward health. When energy is restricted, stagnant, or fragmented, degeneration accelerates.

Energy is not only physical; it is emotional, neurological, and relational. It is influenced by unresolved grief, chronic stress, unexpressed truth, and prolonged inner contraction. People do not lose energy purely through physical exertion. They lose it through internal conflict, fear, rumination, resentment, and emotional suppression. These internal drains are often more exhausting than physical work.

Conscious longevity, therefore, involves learning not

only how to generate energy but how to stop hemorrhaging it through unconscious patterns.

Intention is the organizing intelligence that directs awareness and energy toward a particular pattern of becoming. It is often misunderstood as wishful thinking or rigid goal setting. In its deeper sense, intention is not about force; it is about alignment. It is the inner orientation that quietly guides attention, behavior, emotional tone, and biological response.

The body listens to intention not primarily through words, but through the consistency of your state. An intention to live with vitality becomes biologically meaningful when it is embodied in repeated experiences of coherence, regulation, and conscious choice. Your nervous system learns what you truly intend from how you live, not from what you promise yourself.

When awareness, energy, and intention move in the same direction, the body receives a unified message. When they conflict, the system fragments. Many people intend health but live as if the world is constantly dangerous. They intend rest but maintain constant acceleration. They intend longevity but hold unexamined beliefs about aging that quietly erode vitality.

Conscious longevity begins when these forces come into alignment.

Aging as Repeated Internal Climate

One of the most profound misconceptions about aging is that it is driven primarily by time. In reality, it is strongly influenced by the repetition of internal states over time. The body ages in response to what it repeatedly experiences. When it experiences a sense of danger again and again, it adapts toward protection. When it experiences regulation again and again, it adapts toward restoration.

Time does not age the body in isolation. Experience within time does.

Chronic urgency compresses life force. Chronic fear

constricts circulation. Chronic self-criticism sustains stress chemistry. Chronic emotional suppression restricts breath and limits movement. These patterns gradually carve themselves into tissues, posture, digestion, and hormonal rhythms.

Awareness allows you to witness these internal climates. Energy allows you to feel where flow is restricted or free. Intention allows you to gently reorient those patterns without violence toward yourself.

Conscious longevity does not require the elimination of all challenges. It seeks to prevent challenges from hardening into a permanent physiological state. The body is designed to move through cycles of activation and rest, effort and recovery, exertion and repair. Problems arise not from stress itself, but from stress that is never fully resolved. When the nervous system becomes trapped in activation and does not return to rest, the biological terrain for premature aging is created.

Awareness helps complete the stress cycle by allowing the body to register safety again. Energy rebalances when unresolved states are allowed to move and discharge. Intention stabilizes the new pattern so that regulation, rather than agitation, becomes the norm.

These three – awareness, energy, and intention – form the living engine of conscious longevity. Awareness shows you what is happening. Energy shows you how it feels. Intention influences where it will go next.

When these three move together, the body reorganizes toward coherence. As coherence deepens, subtle biological changes take place. Heart rhythm stabilizes. Cortisol patterns normalize. Sleep becomes more restorative. Digestion becomes more efficient. Inflammatory processes soften. Tissue regeneration improves. Even gene expression begins to reflect a different internal environment. These changes unfold not because you have forced the body to obey, but because you have changed the conditions under which the body lives.

This is the quiet power of conscious longevity. It does not demand heroic feats. It asks for honest presence. It asks you to recognize when you are pushing through fatigue instead of listening to it. It asks you to feel when emotional contraction is shaping your breath. It asks you to notice when your desire for health is being undermined by a pace of living that denies restoration.

Conscious longevity does not demand perfection. It asks for participation.

As you live this way, aging stops feeling like an adversary and begins to feel like a feedback system. Sensations become information rather than threats. Fatigue becomes a teacher instead of a failure. Emotional discomfort becomes a doorway rather than a defect.

This change in relationship dissolves the inner war that quietly accelerates decline. Instead of trying to outrun time, you begin to inhabit it. Instead of resisting change, you begin to collaborate with it. Instead of measuring your life only by what is lost, you begin to recognize what is deepening.

In this way, conscious longevity extends life not just by adding years, but by expanding your capacity to live those years with clarity, resilience, and meaning. The body is no longer a problem to be solved, but a dialogue to be cherished. Awareness keeps the conversation honest. Energy keeps it alive. Intention keeps it oriented toward growth. Together, they form a living practice of conscious longevity.

Breathing Exercise: Activating Coherent Energy

(Approximately five minutes.)

You may wish to explore the following breathing practice to feel how awareness and intention can shape your energy.

Sit upright, or stand with your spine comfortably aligned, and place one hand on your lower abdomen and the other on your chest. Begin by noticing your natural breath for a few moments.

Then inhale through your nose for a slow count of five, allowing the abdomen to expand first and then the chest. Exhale through your mouth for a slow count of seven, allowing the chest to soften first and then the abdomen. Let each exhale become a deliberate release of internal holding.

As you breathe, silently repeat the words "I awaken" on the inhale and "I soften" on the exhale. Continue this rhythm for several minutes. When you feel complete, allow your breath to return to its natural pattern and notice the quality of your internal energy.

Guided Meditation: Aligning Awareness, Energy, and Intention

(Approximately eight to ten minutes.)

Find a comfortable position, either sitting or lying down, and gently close your eyes. Bring your awareness to the sensation of your body breathing. Feel the movement of the breath in your abdomen, your ribs, and your chest. Without trying to change anything, simply notice where your energy feels open and where it feels restricted.

Now, bring to mind one simple intention for your life in this moment – perhaps a sense of wholeness, vitality, peace, or clarity. Choose an intention that feels honest and kind. Allow this intention to rest lightly in your awareness.

Imagine that each inhale draws your energy into alignment with this intention and that each exhale releases anything that interferes with it. There is no strain in this process; there is only gentle orientation. Silently affirm, "My body and my awareness are learning to move together."

Remain here for several breaths, resting inside this alignment. When you are ready, begin to deepen your breathing slightly, notice the support beneath you, and slowly open your eyes, bringing a trace of that alignment into the next moments of your day.

Reflection Prompts

If you wish to integrate these ideas more deeply, you

might take some time to reflect or journal.

You can explore where in your life awareness and intention already feel aligned and where they feel out of sync. You might gently notice where your energy seems to leak away – through worry, overcommitment, self-criticism, or unresolved emotion. You can ask how your nervous system is responding to your current pace of living and whether it feels mostly regulated or frequently overwhelmed. You might become curious about what beliefs you carry about aging and how those beliefs may be shaping your biology. Finally, you can consider what it would mean, in practical and emotional terms, to extend your life not only by adding time but by deepening your presence within it.

Awareness, energy, and intention shape the internal conditions of the body. Yet healing does not occur only within a single layer of experience. Human beings are multidimensional systems in which emotion, biology, memory, and consciousness continuously interact across both visible and invisible planes.

In the next chapter, we move into the multidimensional nature of healing itself – how energy, emotion, and consciousness shape the body across these layers, and how true longevity emerges when healing is allowed to occur across dimensions rather than in isolation.

CHAPTER 8:
WHEN THE SOUL SPEAKS

"When the soul speaks, it does not reveal something new. It reminds us of what we have always known but have long forgotten."
— Maria L. Ellis

There are moments in life when knowledge does not arrive through study, reason, or experience in the outer world, but through a quiet inner encounter that forever changes the way we understand who we are. For me, that moment came not through a teacher, a book, or a scientific discovery, but through a direct and tender conversation with my soul. What unfolded that night reshaped my understanding of time, identity, faith, and purpose. It revealed to me that consciousness does not begin with birth, nor does it end with death – and that the story of who we are is far older, richer, and more sacred than we ever imagine.

When My Soul Remembered

Four lives. Four purposes. One soul. Me.

That evening, the ocean was unusually quiet. The soft rhythm of the waves moved like breath itself – slow, steady, and seemingly infinite. I was alone in my oceanfront apartment, wrapped in the kind of stillness that only arrives when the outer world finally grows quiet enough for the inner world to speak.

I was not seeking visions. I was not asking questions. I was simply reflecting, resting in a peaceful evening and gazing at the darkening horizon where the sea melts into the sky.

That is when I felt my soul. Not as a voice in my ears. Not as a sound in the room. She appeared as a tender knowing that entered my awareness with the gentleness of a whisper and the certainty of truth. Her presence was immediate and unmistakable. I knew her without introduction.

Elianore. My soul.

At one point, I began referring to my soul by name, Elianore, not as a practice I was taught, but as something that emerged naturally, a way of acknowledging the deepest part of myself as a presence rather than an abstraction. She did not feel separate from me, yet she was clearly not the voice of my mind. Her presence felt older than this lifetime, wiser than any personality I had ever worn, and infinitely compassionate. She wrapped around my awareness like a memory I had always carried but had forgotten how to access. I did not see her with my physical eyes. I felt her in the deepest interior of my being.

And then – without warning – she opened the door of remembrance.

Four Lifetimes

The knowing did not arrive as a sequence. It came as a simultaneous unfolding – four lifetimes revealed in a single wave of awareness.

In my First Lifetime, I saw myself in Alexandria, Egypt. I was a scribe.

I loved books with a devotion that felt sacred. I lived inside knowledge. The great Library of Alexandria was not just a place of learning; it felt like the heartbeat of the world. I could sense the texture of parchment under my hands, smell the ink, and feel the vibration of ideas passing through me as I copied and preserved texts.

Then I felt the devastation, the fire, the loss, the burning of the library when the Romans attacked. The grief of watching wisdom turn to ash entered me with a force so real that my chest tightened. In the midst of that pain, Elianore whispered without words: ***This is why you write. This is why only you can write from your perspective. This is why the written word moves your soul so deeply.***

I wept, because suddenly my love for writing was no longer just a gift or a profession. It was the continuation of a vow made across lifetimes.

In my Second Lifetime, my vision shifted. I found myself in the south of France as a medical doctor. I worked with the healing power of plants. I did not rely only on instruments and procedures; I understood the intelligence of nature. Leaves, roots, and flowers were my pharmacy. I felt the reverence I once carried for the remedies of the Earth, for the way life itself could heal when properly guided.

Again, Elianore revealed: ***This is why you are drawn to longevity. This is why you write about health, wellness, and the extension of life through nature, consciousness, and awareness.***

In my Third Lifetime, I was an elder in a village in Peru not a ruler but an advisor. My role was not to command, but to hold wisdom. I sat with other elders. We spoke with patience. We guided the community through seasons of fear and drought, through births and deaths. I could feel the weight of responsibility and the quiet satisfaction of serving the collective good.

Softly, Elianore revealed: ***This is why you counsel. This is why people trust your guidance. This is why leadership feels natural to you.***

In my Fourth Lifetime, I saw myself in another dimension, not on Earth. I was part of a Peace Council. There were no bodies as we understand them here – only presence, intelligence, light, and a profound sense of unity. We did not debate; we harmonized. Our purpose was the preservation of peace across vast systems of life.

From that memory rose the deepest recognition of all.

Once more, Elianore spoke in silence: *This is why you seek peace wherever you go.* **This is why conflict unsettles your soul so deeply. This is why your heart leans naturally toward unity and reconciliation.**

In one wave, I understood that what I loved in this life was not random. It was continuity.

Practice: Feeling the Threads of Continuity

If you wish, you can pause here and gently close your eyes for a moment. Bring to mind three things you have always been drawn to – perhaps writing, healing, teaching, creating, or mediating peace. Let each one appear clearly in your awareness. Then quietly ask yourself: *What if these callings did not begin in this lifetime? What if they are the continuation of something my soul has loved for a very long time?*

Notice how your body responds – not with proof or explanation, but with resonance. Sometimes the soul does not answer in words. It answers in a subtle feeling of "yes" that spreads through the chest, the breath, or the heart.

Fear, Faith, and the Night I Could Not Sleep

The emotional tone of that night was gentle and overwhelming all at once. I felt awe so vast it was like standing before the ocean during a storm: beautiful, powerful, and impossible to ignore. I could not sleep. My mind, shaped by a lifetime of Christian teachings in which past lives were never discussed, struggled to integrate what my soul had revealed.

I had been raised to believe in God, heaven, and eternal life but not in reincarnation, not in lifetimes layered upon one another like sacred chapters of a single eternal book. Fear rose quietly, not fear of Elianore, but fear of what this knowing would mean for everything I thought I understood.

In that trembling place between belief and revelation, I whispered inwardly, "Please only show me what I am able to assimilate." Elianore answered with the gentlest assurance I have ever known: *You are safe. You are loved. You are protected.*

The fear softened immediately. It was not erased, but it was held.

My curiosity then turned toward the future. I was afraid to look too far. I did not want to know the exact moment of my death or the details of how my life would end. I asked only to glimpse five years ahead. Then, gathering courage, I chose to see ten years – to age eighty-five, and no more.

In that moment, I understood something essential: the soul does not measure time the way we do. The soul is time-less. The soul walks beside us through every lifetime.

Elianore also clarified something that healed the seeming conflict between my Christian faith and this revelation. She revealed that God is above us: the infinite divine intelligence. The spirit is the breath that animates the body. **The soul is the eternal self-traveling through lifetimes. There was no contradiction. There was completion.**

The Confidence That Was Born That Night

This experience did not make me more uncertain. It made me more confident than I had ever been. I have always seen myself as a confident woman, but this knowing reshaped confidence into something much deeper. It was no longer built on personality, success, intellect, or accomplishment. It was anchored in identity beyond time.

I trusted myself even more after that night, because I finally understood who I was beneath the roles, the professions, and the timelines. I knew I was not merely a body moving into the later seasons of life. I was an eternal soul evolving through form.

My fear of death dissolved quietly and completely. I no longer see death as an ending. I see it as a transition of consciousness. We do not come to Earth to finish. We come to learn, evolve, remember, and exercise free will. Longevity, then, is not only about extending the life of the body. It is about deepening the soul's curriculum within each lifetime.

From that night forward, I no longer walked alone. I felt accompanied at the deepest level of being. Decisions felt different. Fear held less power. Aging felt less threatening. Purpose felt clearer.

I now understood that everything I had loved in this life – writing, healing, leading, mentoring, seeking peace – was not random. It was continuity, memory written into the soul. I realized that we are not born blank. We arrive with memories woven into our essence. We remember not with the mind alone, but with resonance. That night with Elianore did not separate me from the world. It rooted me more fully within it.

Breathing Exercise: Remembering the Eternal Self

(Approximately five minutes.)

You may wish to explore a simple breath practice to anchor this awareness in your body.

Find a quiet place where you can sit comfortably upright. Allow your shoulders to soften and your hands to rest gently where they feel most natural. Begin to inhale slowly through your nose for a count of five, feeling your chest and abdomen expand with air. Then exhale softly through your mouth for a count of seven, allowing your body to relax more fully with each out breath.

As you inhale, you can silently repeat the phrase, "I welcome my eternal self." As you exhale, you can gently affirm, "I release fear of time." Continue in this way for several minutes, letting the rhythm of your breath become smooth and unhurried. When you feel complete, allow your breathing to return to its natural pattern and notice how you feel – perhaps slightly more spacious, more grounded, or quietly reassured.

Let your breath remind you that you are more than a single moment in time.

Guided Meditation: Meeting Your Soul

(Approximately eight to ten minutes.)

If you wish to deepen your connection with the soul, you can explore this guided meditation.

Close your eyes and first notice the quiet inside your chest. Bring your attention gently to the center of your heart. Allow your breath to move in and out without effort, as if the body is breathing itself.

Now imagine a soft light rising gently from within – not from outside you, but from the deepest center of your being. This light does not need to be bright or dramatic. It may feel warm, subtle, or simply peaceful. Let this light represent your soul.

You do not need to "see" anything clearly. It is enough to sense the presence of this inner light. When you feel ready, you may ask silently within, "What do you want me to remember?" Do not force an answer. Simply allow impressions, feelings, images, or a sense of quiet peace to arise.

You may notice only a subtle shift, a feeling of being more held or more known. Trust that this, too, is communication. Rest here for several minutes, letting yourself be in gentle contact with this inner presence.

Before returning, you might affirm inwardly, "I trust the wisdom that lives within me." When you are ready, bring your awareness back to the room. Feel your body, the support beneath you, and the sounds around you. Then gently open your eyes, carrying a trace of that connection into your next moments.

Reflection Prompts

If you wish to integrate this chapter more fully, you may spend time journaling or quietly contemplating a few questions.

You might reflect on whether you have ever felt guided by something deeper than your rational mind, perhaps in decisions that turned out to be wiser than you could logically explain. You can explore which lifelong patterns or callings feel as though they might come from a deeper source — those interests or talents that have been part of you for as long as you can remember.

You may consider how your relationship with aging would change if you truly believed your soul was eternal, and what fears might soften if you trusted that consciousness continues beyond this body. Finally, you might ask yourself: if my soul were to speak to me tonight, what would I hope it would say, and what reassurance or guidance would I most want to receive?

That night, alone beside the ocean, I did not lose my faith. I expanded it. I did not abandon God. I understood God more fully. I did not become less human. I remembered that I am more than human. Elianore walks with me now — not as a distant mystery, but as an intimate companion in every breath, every choice, and every future remembrance. And this is why I know, without doubt, that longevity is not only biological. It is eternal.

CHAPTER 9:
THE MULTIDIMENSIONAL SOUL: HOW AWARENESS TRAVELS ACROSS LIFETIMES, DIMENSIONS, AND STATES OF BEING

"You are not a drop in the ocean.
You are the entire ocean in a drop."

— Rumi

As consciousness deepens and healing begins to unfold across dimensions, a natural question arises: *What is it that is aware?* If the body responds to emotion, memory, and meaning — and if awareness can observe and integrate all three — then what is the deeper continuity that moves through these layers? What is this presence that watches the changing body, the shifting feelings, and the evolving story, yet somehow remains?

The First Time I Felt the Soul Was Larger Than This Lifetime

For much of my life, I thought of the soul as something abstract — beautiful and meaningful, but distant. I believed I *had* a soul, but I did not yet know what it meant to experience myself *as* soul.

That understanding did not arrive through study or

101

belief. It came through a quiet, undeniable feeling that changed me forever. It unfolded during a season when I was spending more time in stillness than at any other time in my life. My days had slowed. My body was calmer. My nervous system had begun to trust rest. In that softened state, something within me became more open – less defended, less hurried.

One evening, as I sat alone in the quiet after a long day, I slipped into stillness without effort. My breathing slowed on its own. My thoughts thinned. I no longer felt as though I was trying to meditate. I simply was. Then, without warning, I felt myself expand – not physically, not emotionally, but in a way that ordinary language cannot easily capture.

It was as though the edges of the person I had always believed myself to be gently dissolved. I was still Maria, still sitting in the room, yet at the same time I felt vast – far larger than memory, far larger than personality, far larger than this single life story. There was no fear in this experience, only a deep familiarity. It felt like remembering something I had always known and had quietly forgotten.

In that moment, I did not feel bound to my age. I did not feel bound to my history. I did not feel bound to time at all. I felt like awareness itself – watching, resting, existing without effort. When the sensation gradually softened and I returned fully to ordinary perception, I opened my eyes and remained very still. My heart was steady. My body was calm. But inside, something fundamental had shifted.

For the first time in my life, I did not simply *believe* that the soul was multidimensional. I felt it as truth.

From that day forward, the fear of time began to loosen its grip. Aging no longer felt like a narrowing corridor. Death no longer felt like disappearance. Life felt like a continuum rather than a single chapter.

This realization changed how I understood suffering as well. I had always thought of pain as belonging solely to this life, this story. Now, I began to sense that pain, like wisdom, travels through layers of awareness deeper than personality alone. It is carried, transformed, and sometimes resolved across dimensions of experience I do not yet fully comprehend. This understanding did not make life less precious. It made it more meaningful.

Months later, another moment deepened this knowing. I was holding the hand of someone I loved who was suffering. As I sat beside them in silence, a tender calm settled over me. I suddenly sensed that I was not witnessing only a physical struggle. I was witnessing a soul passing through a profound threshold of experience.

Again, without words, I felt it: this life was not the entire story. It was a single passage within a much greater symphony. That awareness did not remove the grief, but it changed its texture. Loss no longer felt like annihilation. It felt like transition. Around this time, I noticed memories and inner impressions that did not seem anchored only in this lifetime – sudden feelings of familiarity in places I had never visited, deep emotional recognition with people I had only just met, longings that did not appear to arise from my personal history. Rather than dismissing these as imagination, I began to hold them gently as possible whispers from deeper layers of awareness.

I no longer felt compelled to define them. I simply listened.

As this awareness grew, I started to feel the difference between consciousness and the soul. Consciousness felt like the light that witnesses. The soul felt like the journey of that light across experience. My body felt like the vessel for this journey – not its source.

My identity softened. I experienced myself not only as a woman with a particular life story, but as awareness moving through that story. This shift transformed my relationship with fear. Rather than registering solely as a signal of danger, fear often appeared as resistance to remembering what I already was.

When fear appeared, I began to meet it with curiosity instead of panic. I asked, *What part of me feels threatened, and what part of me remains untouched by this?* Every time, I discovered a presence within me that stayed vast, quiet, and unchanged.

One night, this understanding became especially vivid. I woke from a dream with the feeling that I had been somewhere beyond form and language. I could not describe what I had seen, but I knew what I had felt – an infinite tenderness, a natural order without rigidity, a presence that was both intimate and immense.

As I lay there in the dark, I realized something that took my breath away: I had not dreamed of *another place*. I had remembered another aspect of myself.

From that moment on, I stopped thinking of life as a line moving from beginning to end. I began to experience it as a multi-layered unfolding, where awareness moves through bodies, emotions, and dimensions with far more freedom than the personality can understand.

The soul no longer felt theoretical. It felt personal, present, and continuous. This did not pull me away from my human life. It anchored me more deeply within it. I loved it more freely. I feared less intensely. I am aged with less resistance. I lived with greater tenderness toward myself and others.

Knowing that I was more than this body did not make the body less sacred. It made it a sacred, temporary home for an eternal traveler. In that knowing, longevity transformed once again. It was no longer simply about extending the life of the body. It became about honoring the soul's journey through every stage of being – this lifetime included.

I was not passing through life toward disappearance. I was traveling through life as consciousness itself – learning, remembering, and expanding. For the first time, the mystery of existence did not frighten me. It felt like home.

Mini-Practice: Touching the Continuity of Awareness

If you feel called, you can pause for a brief experiment. Let your eyes soften or close. Bring to mind a memory from childhood – perhaps a moment in a classroom, a place you played, or a person you loved. Notice the image or feeling of that younger self. Then gently ask, *Who was aware back then?*

Now bring your attention back to this moment, to your breath and your body as they are now. Ask again, *Who is aware right now?* You may notice that while the body, circumstances, and roles have changed, the simple knowing presence that witnesses them feels strangely the same. This quiet continuity is one way the multidimensional soul reveals itself.

The Soul as Continuity of Awareness

For much of modern history, the soul has been treated either as a religious notion or dismissed entirely from scientific conversation. Yet as studies of consciousness grow, and as near-death research, psychophysiology, and trauma science converge, the language of the soul is quietly returning – this time not as rigid doctrine, but as lived experience.

In the context of conscious longevity, the soul is not an abstract idea. It is the inner continuity of awareness that persists through change – the awareness that remains through the changing body, the changing personality, and the changing seasons of life. It is the witnessing presence that remains even as everything else evolves.

You have already known your soul through moments rather than definitions. You have felt it in deep love that seemed to exist beyond logic. You have sensed it in sudden clarity that did not come from analysis. You have touched it in grief that felt larger than the mind could hold. You have recognized it in awe, beauty, longing, and the mysterious feeling of remembrance.

The soul is not separate from the body, but it is not limited to it. It expresses itself through sensation, emotions, intuition, and choice. It animates biological form while also extending beyond it. This is what makes the soul multidimensional.

Human beings do not exist in only one dimension of experience. We live simultaneously as physical organisms, emotional beings, psychological identities, and fields of awareness. The soul is the thread that weaves these dimensions together across time.

When we speak of awareness traveling across lifetimes or dimensions, we are not necessarily describing literal maps and locations. We are pointing toward continuity of consciousness – the way experience seems to carry memory, pattern, and trajectory beyond a single moment, and perhaps beyond a single incarnation.

Many cultures across history have understood life in this way. Indigenous traditions, Eastern philosophies, mystical branches of Christianity, and ancient Egyptian teachings all describe the soul as a traveler moving through phases, realms, and states of being in a long arc of learning and remembrance.

Modern science, while cautious with metaphysical language, is beginning to encounter phenomena that echo these ancient perspectives. Near-death experiences, shared death experiences, spontaneous recall of apparent past-life memories in children, and evidence of awareness persisting beyond measurable brain activity all challenge the assumption that consciousness is created solely by the brain.

Conscious longevity does not ask you to accept any single explanation. It invites you to hold these possibilities with humility and openness, allowing your understanding of what it means to be human to widen.

In this expanded view, the soul is not confined to chronological time. It is not governed solely by birth and death. It moves through states of being in ways that are not linear. It gathers experience, meaning, and memory across dimensions of existence that ordinary waking consciousness perceives only partially.

This understanding redefines the meaning of a single lifetime. Your life becomes not a solitary event racing toward an end, but a chapter within a much larger continuum. Your struggles are not merely obstacles; they are part of an evolving narrative of becoming. Your longings are not random; they may be echoes of a deeper remembrance. Your sense of purpose may not have begun with this body – and may not end with it.

From the perspective of conscious longevity, this has profound implications. If the soul is multidimensional, then aging is not merely the wearing down of matter. It is the ripening of experience. The body may change, but awareness can deepen. The personality may soften, but the soul may grow more luminous. The physical form may slow, but the inner field may widen.

Longevity becomes more than survival. It becomes the conscious participation in a long unfolding of awareness.

You do not need to adopt any particular metaphysical doctrine to relate to this. You need only consider the possibility that your awareness is larger than your current identity.

Even within a single lifetime, you already experience multiple states of being. You move through waking consciousness, dreams, deep sleep, intuitive insight, emotional immersion, meditative stillness, and moments of transcendent clarity. Your awareness does not vanish between these states. It shifts its focus.

At a minimum, the multidimensional soul can be understood as the awareness that travels through these inner worlds, moving across layers of perception without being confined to any one of them.

Trauma research confirms that memory can live outside conscious recall, stored in the body and nervous system. Spiritual traditions suggest that memory may also exist beyond the body. At both the neurological and metaphysical levels, experience appears to travel in ways that the conscious mind alone does not fully control.

What This Means for Healing and Aging

If the soul is multidimensional, then healing is also multidimensional. Healing does not address only the present moment. It can touch unresolved layers of experience that reach far beyond conscious memory. Emotional reactions that feel disproportionate may be rooted in deeper somatic or even layers of self beyond the personal. Long-standing fears, affinities, or callings may not originate solely in this lifetime.

Conscious longevity does not require you to explain these mysteries. It asks only that you respect the depth of the human system.

Treating only the surface layer of experience leaves deeper currents untouched. When awareness, safety, and compassion are allowed into the deeper strata of being, healing often unfolds in ways that appear almost effortless. The soul does not heal through force. It heals through remembrance and integration.

One of the greatest sources of human suffering is the belief that life is fundamentally random and that the self is isolated in an indifferent universe. This belief shrinks meaning and contracts awareness. The recognition of a multidimensional soul reframes existence as participatory rather than accidental. It suggests that life is not merely happening *to* you; it unfolds through you.

This reframing alone alters the biology of hope. Hope is not just emotional optimism. It is a neurochemical state that reorganizes immune function, cellular repair, and hormonal balance. When the nervous system perceives life as meaningful rather than arbitrary, it behaves differently. It invests differently in survival and renewal.

Seeing yourself as a soul traveling through dimensions rather than as a body racing toward decline quiets existential fear. Fear is one of the most powerful accelerants of aging. As fear loosens, energy that was locked in vigilance becomes available for restoration.

The awareness of the soul does not pull you out of life. It anchors you more deeply within it. You stop living as though every moment must be defended. You begin to live as though every moment is part of a larger unfolding that you can participate in consciously.

The multidimensional soul also reframes death — not as annihilation, but as transition. Even if you do not personally accept literal continuation beyond physical life, the psychological and spiritual effect of this perspective is significant. When the terror of extinction softens, the nervous system relaxes. When the panic of finality eases, the body steps out of chronic urgency. Urgency ages the body faster than time itself. Conscious longevity is therefore not only the art of adding years. It is the art of releasing invisible pressures that compress life from within.

When you live from awareness of the multidimensional soul, your experience of time changes. You no longer rush through moments as if they are vanishing forever. You inhabit them as meaningful expressions within a vast continuum. Presence deepens. Attachment loosens. Gratitude grows stronger than fear.

The soul does not measure life by the clock. It measures life by depth of experience. From this perspective, aging is not the loss of youth but the accumulation of meaning. Wrinkles become maps of laughter and sorrow. Time becomes a teacher rather than a thief.

Even suffering takes on a different quality. When seen only through the lens of survival, suffering feels purely punitive. When seen through the lens of soul growth, it becomes intelligible — not easier, but more understandable within a larger context.

This does not romanticize pain. It contextualizes it. The multidimensional soul invites you to view your life as a curriculum of awakening rather than as a series of random events. It invites you to see your body not as a disposable shell, but as a sacred instrument through which awareness learns and expresses itself.

This perspective quietly transforms how you care for yourself. You begin to treat your body with reverence instead of impatience. You begin to nourish your energy rather than spend it carelessly. You begin to listen more deeply to intuition, not as fantasy, but as the language of multidimensional awareness speaking across layers of being.

Conscious longevity, at this level, is not about defeating aging. It is about honoring the vehicle through which the soul continues its journey.

The more you recognize yourself as multidimensional, the less confined you feel by circumstance. Even limitation is held within a wider context. Even decline becomes part of a larger arc of becoming. The fear of being "used up" begins to dissolve. You no longer live as a resource that will soon be depleted. You live as awareness that continues to evolve.

This does not remove the grief of aging. It gives grief a place to belong within meaning rather than isolation. The multidimensional soul holds both the tenderness of impermanence and the stability of continuity. It allows you to love the body without clinging to it. It allows you to grieve loss without believing that loss is the end of meaning.

In this way, the soul becomes a bridge between time and eternity, between biology and mystery, between what can be measured and what can only be deeply known. To age consciously is ultimately to remember who you are beneath form.

And remembrance is one of the most powerful medicines we possess.

Breathing Exercise: Grounding the Multidimensional Self

(Approximately five minutes.)

If you wish to ground this understanding in your body, you can explore the following simple breath practice.

Sit comfortably with your feet resting flat on the floor

and allow your spine to lengthen naturally without strain. Inhale slowly through your nose for a count of five, feeling the breath fill your body. Exhale slowly through your mouth for a count of seven, allowing your shoulders, jaw, and chest to soften.

As you inhale, silently repeat the phrase, "I am present." As you exhale, silently repeat, "I am more than this moment." Let both truths coexist: the solidity of your body and the spaciousness of your awareness. Continue for several minutes. When you are ready, allow your breathing to return to its natural rhythm and notice the sense of grounded presence that remains.

Guided Meditation: Remembering the Multidimensional Soul

(Approximately eight to ten minutes.)

Find a comfortable position and gently close your eyes. Bring your awareness first to your physical body seated in space. Feel the weight of your body and the contact with the chair, cushion, or floor. Allow yourself to truly arrive.

Now, without effort, allow your awareness to gently expand beyond the outline of your physical form. Sense yourself not only as a body, but as a field of perception that extends outward. There is no need to imagine anything dramatic. Simply feel that your presence is slightly wider than your skin.

Silently ask within, "What part of me has been aware my entire life?" Do not search for an intellectual answer. Instead, sense the continuity beneath changing memories, sensations, and roles – the same basic "I am" that was present in childhood, adolescence, adulthood, and this moment now.

Rest as that awareness for several breaths. Let it feel simple, natural, and unforced. Then, softly affirm to yourself, "I am carried by a consciousness larger than my fear." Allow these words to settle gently within you.

When you are ready, bring your attention back into your

physical body, feel the support beneath you, notice the sounds around you, and slowly open your eyes, bringing a trace of this remembering into your day.

Reflection Prompts

If you would like to deepen your relationship with this chapter, you might spend time reflecting or journaling.

You can recall moments in your life when you sensed that you were more than your physical body – perhaps through love, loss, synchronicity, or timeless presence. You might explore how viewing yourself as a multidimensional being changes the way you relate to aging. You can notice which fears begin to soften when you consider life as a continuum rather than a one-time event. You may look at your current challenges through the lens of soul growth and ask what they might be teaching you at a deeper level. Finally, you might consider what it would mean to live as a remembering soul rather than a racing personality in your daily choices, relationships, and self-care.

As awareness of the multidimensional soul deepens, another question naturally arises: if the soul travels and evolves across dimensions, does it follow a deeper design or pattern of purpose?

In the next chapter, we explore the concept of the soul's blueprint – how meaning, destiny, and deeper soul patterns may shape the arc of human life, and how conscious longevity unfolds when we align with that deeper design.

CHAPTER 10:
CONSCIOUS LIVING PRACTICES: A DAILY BLUEPRINT FOR LONGEVITY AND AWAKENING

"How we spend our days is, of course, how we spend our lives."
— Annie Dillard

Awareness changes everything – but awareness alone is not enough. What reshapes the body, rewires the nervous system, and transforms the trajectory of aging is how awareness is translated into daily living. Conscious longevity is not built in moments of insight alone. It is built through the small, repeated choices of ordinary days.

Many people assume that transformation requires dramatic change. In truth, it is the subtle, consistent recalibration of daily life that quietly restructures the internal environment of the body and the consciousness that lives within it. The body does not change because of grand intentions. The body does not change through grand intentions alone; it changes through rhythm, repetition, and relationship with the body.

Conscious living is the bridge between understanding and embodiment. It is how the insights of awareness touch the nervous system, the hormonal system, the immune system, and the emotional life. Without conscious daily practices, even the most profound realizations remain abstract. With them, the body learns a new way of being.

How My Ordinary Days Became the Practice

For a long time, I believed that transformation required extraordinary moments – retreats, breakthroughs, crises, or profound spiritual experiences. I assumed awakening would arrive in waves of revelation. What I did not understand was that the deepest change would come quietly, disguised as routine.

It began not with a vision, but with a small decision I made one morning. Instead of reaching for my phone the moment I woke up, I sat at the edge of the bed and placed my feet on the floor. I took one slow breath. Then another. I placed my hand over my heart and asked, "How do I feel right now?" The question startled me with its intimacy.

I realized that for years, I had been waking up and immediately running into schedules, expectations, responsibilities, and noise – without ever checking in with the body that carried me through all of it. That morning, for the first time in a long while, I didn't rush past myself. It seemed like a small act, almost insignificant, yet something had shifted. That single pause became the beginning of a new way of living.

At first, I practiced awareness clumsily. I would remember to slow my breathing halfway through a stressful conversation. I would notice tension only after my shoulders had been tight for hours. I would forget to be present, and then gently begin again without punishing myself. What surprised me most was how forgiving the body was. It did not demand perfection. It responded with gratitude to even the smallest moments of attention.

As days turned into weeks, something remarkable unfolded. My rituals did not look dramatic from the outside. I drank water more slowly. I walked with intention instead of rushing. I paused before eating. I learned to sense when my system was nearing overload and, instead of pushing through, I rested.

For most of my life, rest had felt like weakness. Now, it felt like intelligence.

I began to see how deeply I had been living in reaction rather than in choice. My habits had been shaped by urgency instead of alignment. I worked when I was exhausted. I ate when I was distracted. I listened while preparing my response. My life had been efficient, but it had not been coherent. Conscious living asked something radically different of me. It asked me to become present for my life.

The real awakening did not occur only in silence or meditation. It unfolded in traffic, grocery aisles, difficult conversations, and quiet evenings at home. I began to notice how often my breath tightened in moments of uncertainty, and how quickly I left my body to attend to others. Slowly, gently, I learned to stay.

One afternoon, I caught myself in the middle of an old pattern – rushing through a task, jaw tense, mind already leaping ahead. I stopped. I exhaled. I softened my face. I continued what I was doing, but from a different state. That was one of the first times I realized that daily life itself had become my practice. I was no longer waiting for sacred moments. I was allowing ordinary moments to become sacred.

The most powerful shift came when I began to listen to my energy instead of overriding it. I learned the difference between tiredness that was asking for rest and resistance that was asking for presence. I discovered that slowing down did not make me less effective; it made me more accurate and more honest.

I also noticed something profound: my body began to change in response to my choices. My sleep deepened. My digestion improved. My immune system felt stronger. Pain I had accepted as "normal aging" softened without any aggressive intervention. I had not altered my genes. I had changed my relationship with my nervous system.

Conscious living was not about doing more. It was about doing less in conflict with myself.

There was one evening that marked a turning point. I had just finished a long day and felt the familiar pull to distract myself – to numb out with a screen or drift into endless scrolling. Instead, I lit a candle and sat quietly at the table. I placed both feet on the floor and allowed my breathing to slow. In that stillness, I realized something unexpected. I wasn't truly tired. I was overstimulated. For years, I had confused those two states.

As my nervous system began to settle, a quiet aliveness returned – not the adrenaline of productivity, but the warmth of presence. In that warmth, I felt an unfamiliar emotion rise to the surface: contentment. Not accomplishment. Not relief. Not distraction. Contentment.

In that moment, I understood that longevity is not only preserved through medicine and supplements. It is preserved through the way we live our minutes, not just our years.

From that night forward, I made a simple commitment: I would no longer live as if rest, breath, and presence were rewards to be earned after everything else was finished. They would become foundational.

My days changed shape – not so much outwardly, but inwardly. I still worked. I still cared for others. I still met obligations. But I began to do all of these things differently. I learned to begin my mornings in coherence rather than reactivity, and I let my emotions move through me instead of storing them quietly in my body. **Most importantly, I came to see that longevity is not created by bursts of intensity. It is created through the quiet consistency of conscious living.**

The awakening I once imagined as dramatic turned out to be far more intimate. It was woven into the way I stood at the kitchen sink, the way I listened when someone spoke, the way I responded to my fatigue, and the way I honored my breath when no one was watching.

My life did not become easier. It became truer. And in that truth, something remarkable occurred: I began to feel younger. Not because time had reversed, but because my relationship with time had softened. That is when I understood that conscious living is not a phase or a trend. It is a daily blueprint for awakening, built one ordinary, intentional choice at a time.

Practice: A Morning Check-In

(Thirty to forty-five seconds.)

You may wish to try the same experiment.

Tomorrow morning, before you reach for your phone or step into your day, sit at the edge of your bed with your feet on the floor. Take one slow breath in through your nose and one slow breath out through your mouth. Place your hand over your heart and quietly ask yourself, "How do I feel right now?" Do not try to fix anything. Simply listen for a few moments. This is how ordinary time becomes sacred — not by changing what you do, but by changing how you arrive.

The Foundations of Conscious Living

A conscious living practice is not a rigid routine. It is a living relationship with your life that is rooted in presence. Each day, it asks a simple but powerful question: How am I relating to my body, my time, my emotions, my energy, and my sense of meaning right now?

Longevity is not created by isolated behaviors. It is shaped by the overall climate in which those behaviors occur. A perfectly designed diet practiced in a state of constant stress will not produce the same biological outcome as a simpler diet lived in a state of coherence and connection. Exercise done with self-judgment does not create the same physiology as movement done with appreciation. Sleep achieved under pressure does not restore the same way as sleep entered through a regulated nervous system.

For this reason, conscious living is not about optimization alone. It is about alignment.

Your nervous system is constantly asking whether life

feels safe, coherent, and meaningful. When those conditions are present, the body naturally shifts from defense into regeneration. When they are absent, the body remains in survival mode, even if everything looks "fine" from the outside.

Daily conscious practices teach the body that safety and meaning can be consistent rather than rare. One common misunderstanding of modern wellness culture is the belief that the body can be forced into health through discipline alone. Discipline has its place, but the body ultimately responds more deeply to relationship than to rules. It listens not only to what you do but to how you do it – your emotional tone, your nervous system state, and your inner dialogue as you act.

Conscious living begins with rhythm rather than control. It invites you to listen before you impose. It invites collaboration with your body rather than conquest. It invites you to see your daily life not as something to get through, but as the primary field in which longevity and awakening are cultivated.

The blueprint for conscious living rests on a handful of foundational relationships: your relationship with breath, with rest, with movement, with nourishment, with emotion, with attention, and with meaning. These are not separate categories; together they form a single interwoven system.

Your breath is not simply a mechanical exchange of oxygen and carbon dioxide. It is the fastest and most reliable way to regulate the nervous system. Every breath shapes heart rhythm, vagal tone, and emotional state. The way you breathe throughout the day quietly sets the internal tempo of your biology.

Rest is not the absence of productivity. It is an active biological process of repair. Without sufficient rest, the body cannot complete the cycles of regeneration that extend functional lifespan. Chronic fatigue is often not a sign of inadequacy; it is a signal that the body has been living too long without enough coherence and restoration.

Movement is not punishment for the body. It is communication with it. When movement is approached as collaboration rather than correction, it restores circulation, supports lymphatic flow, and integrates neural pathways. The body thrives on movement that feels kind, rhythmic, and alive.

Nourishment is more than chemistry; it is signaling. What and how you eat conveys messages of safety, scarcity, pleasure, or punishment to the nervous system. Eating in a state of presence and appreciation influences digestion, hormone balance, and metabolic efficiency.

Emotion is not an interruption of biology; it is one of its architects. Suppressed emotion does not disappear; it settles into the tissues, the breath, and the posture of the body. Over time, chronic emotional contraction shapes the way we stand, breathe, and respond to life. Conscious living creates space for emotion to be felt, acknowledged, and integrated.

Attention is one of the most potent regulators of physiology. Where attention goes, neural resources follow. A life lived in continuous distraction fragments the nervous system, while a life that includes moments of sustained, gentle attention stabilizes it.

Meaning is not a philosophical luxury; it is a biological resource. People who experience a sense of meaning tend to live longer, recover more quickly, and show greater resilience in illness. The body needs purpose as deeply as it needs nutrients.

These relationships form the living architecture of conscious longevity. No single practice transforms the body on its own; it is the coherence between them that reshapes the internal environment in which aging unfolds.

For this reason, conscious living is not about perfection; it is about noticing. It is about returning again and again to the present moment and asking what alignment looks like now – not yesterday, not ideally, not someday, but now.

Many people try to live consciously by adding more to

already crowded lives: more tasks, more practices, more pressure to "do it right." In reality, conscious living tends to simplify rather than complicate. It gently removes what is no longer aligned and strengthens what is already life-giving.

One of the most radical acts of conscious living is learning to slow down without collapsing. Slowing down allows the nervous system to exit perpetual urgency. It allows the body to complete its natural repair cycles. It allows emotions to surface without being immediately pushed aside. It creates space for meaning to be felt, not just thought about.

The pace at which you live shapes the pace at which your cells age.

Another essential practice is self-observation without judgment. Many people relate to themselves through criticism, urgency, or endless expectation. Conscious living introduces a different relationship: one of curiosity. Curiosity relaxes the nervous system, while judgment tightens it. The body cannot easily regenerate in an environment of constant internal threat.

When you observe yourself gently, you begin to see patterns not as failures but as information. You notice how stress enters your body, how fatigue accumulates, how certain interactions affect your energy, and how old beliefs quietly shape your choices. This awareness is not meant to shame you into change; it is meant to invite collaboration.

As time passes, conscious living begins to reshape identity itself. You no longer define yourself primarily by what you produce, endure, or control. You begin to define yourself by how you relate, how you listen, how you align with your truth, and how you participate in your unfolding.

As identity shifts, the body responds. Hormonal patterns stabilize. Sleep becomes more restorative. Inflammation quiets. Emotional regulation becomes more stable. The subtle sense of being at war with time begins to dissolve.

In this framework, longevity is no longer a race against aging; it is a partnership with life.

The simplicity of conscious living can feel almost

unsettling in a culture attached to complexity. It does not ask you to conquer your biology but to befriend it. It does not ask you to overpower your nervous system but to regulate it. It does not ask you to chase meaning but to notice where meaning already lives.

Ultimately, conscious living invites you to remember a fundamental truth: your body is not only a structure of cells; it is a listener. It is listening to the way you speak to yourself. It is listening to what you believe about aging, safety, worth, and time. And it responds accordingly.

Conscious living becomes a form of biological communication. Every small act of presence sends a message of coherence. Every moment of regulation sends a message of safety. Every experience of meaning sends a message of vitality. Over months and years, these messages quietly reshape how the body ages.

This is not a quick intervention. It is a lifelong conversation. But it is a conversation whose effects accumulate in powerful and often beautiful ways.

A daily blueprint for conscious living does not require rigid scheduling. It requires remembering, again and again, that your life is not happening outside of you; it is happening through you. The quality of that experience is shaping the biology that carries you forward.

Daily Blueprint for Conscious Longevity

Below is a practical structure that allows every reader to succeed. Whether someone has five minutes or nearly an hour, they can live a day anchored in conscious longevity. The goal is not to complete every step; it is to support the three relationships daily in ways that feel attainable.

The Essential Day: Five Minutes

A day where you do the least, but it still counts.

One Minute for the Body:

Place your feet on the ground, inhale slowly, and scan

your body from head to toe. Notice without judgment. Acknowledge one sensation.

Two Minutes for the Mind:

Close your eyes, inhale through the nose, exhale through the mouth, and observe your thoughts as if they were clouds moving across the sky. You do not need to change anything; simply witness.

Two minutes for Meaning:

Ask yourself one question: *What matters most to me today?*

Choose a single guiding intention and carry it gently into your day.

Even when life feels overwhelming, these five minutes anchor you back into coherence.

Solid Day: Fifteen to Twenty Minutes

A grounded, supportive day for the average busy person.

Five Minutes for the Body:

Breathe deeply and stretch your spine, neck, and shoulders. Place one hand on your heart and one on your abdomen, and breathe until both move rhythmically.

Five Minutes for the Mind:

Practice a simple centering meditation. Inhale and silently say, "I am here." Exhale and silently say, "I am safe." Repeat until your thoughts slow to a gentle pace.

Five to Ten Minutes for Meaning:

Write a brief reflection.

What is one quality you choose to embody today: presence, patience, courage, or compassion? Let it guide how you move, listen, and respond.

What is one habit, belief, or tension you are willing to release – urgency, self-judgment, or the need to control? Notice how space opens when you no longer carry it.

Even small, conscious choices shape the tone of the day

– and over time, the direction of a life.

What is one thing you want to move toward?

This creates emotional coherence – a state where the mind and body work together rather than in conflict.

Ideal Day: Thirty to Forty-Five Minutes

*A fully supportive day that nourishes
all aspects of conscious longevity.*

Ten Minutes for the Body:

Begin with slow joint rotations, gentle stretches, or mindful walking – enough to awaken circulation and bring you into your physical presence. Follow with three slow, diaphragmatic breaths with your hands over your chest and belly.

Ten to Fifteen Minutes for the Mind:

Sit in quiet meditation. Practice observing your thoughts without attachment. Bring attention to your breath, your heart rhythm, or the sensation of the present moment. Allow your awareness to expand beyond your physical boundaries.

Ten to Twenty Minutes for Meaning:

Engage in reflective or creative practice. Journal. Pray. Read something uplifting. Write a single sentence of gratitude. Visualize the kind of person you are becoming. Connect with purpose, not performance.

The ideal day does not demand perfection. It offers space – space for awareness, renewal, and alignment.

When you nurture the body, the mind, and meaning – even briefly – you change the entire trajectory of your day. Over time, these moments accumulate into a new way of living. Longevity is not built in dramatic moments. It is built in the quiet ones. The blueprint is simple, but the impact is profound.

Breathing Exercise: The Breath of Daily Regulation

(Approximately five minutes.)

You may wish to explore the following practice as a simple daily anchor.

Sit comfortably with both feet resting on the ground. Allow your spine to rise naturally without strain. Inhale through your nose for a slow count of four. Exhale gently through your mouth for a slow count of six, letting each exhale be slightly longer and softer than the inhale.

As you breathe, silently repeat the phrase "I receive" on the inhale and "I release" on the exhale. Feel the body subtly settling with each breath. After several minutes, allow your breath to return to its natural rhythm and notice any shifts in your internal state.

Guided Meditation: Living From Alignment

(Approximately eight to ten minutes.)

Find a comfortable position and gently close your eyes. Bring your attention to the natural rhythm of your breath and feel the gentle rise and fall of your body.

Begin by bringing awareness to the rhythm of your day: how you wake, how you move, how you work, how you rest. Without criticism, simply sense how your daily life feels inside your body.

Quietly ask within, "Where in my life do I feel aligned?" Allow any sensation, memory, or awareness to arise. Then ask, "Where in my life do I feel strained or hurried?" Again, simply notice what appears, trusting that noticing is enough for now.

As you continue to breathe, imagine that your breath moves gently into the areas of strain, creating space there. With each exhale, imagine those areas softening slightly. Silently affirm, "I am allowed to live in rhythm."

Remain here for several more breaths. When you feel ready, begin to deepen your breathing. Notice the support beneath you and the sounds around you. Slowly open your eyes, carrying a sense of alignment forward into your day.

Reflection Prompts

You may find it nourishing to reflect or journal on questions such as these:

- Where in your daily life do you feel most aligned with yourself?
- Where do you feel the greatest sense of strain, urgency, or fragmentation?
- How does your current pace of life affect your body and your emotions?
- What small, realistic daily shift would most support your sense of coherence right now?
- What does "conscious living" mean to you in practical terms at this stage of your life?

Daily conscious practices steadily regulate the internal environment of the body. Yet beneath these practices lies an even deeper reality: a vast, invisible field in which matter, energy, and awareness arise together.

In the next chapter, we move beyond the personal and into the universal. We explore the field in which consciousness becomes reality itself, where science begins to touch spirit, and where the deeper architecture of existence quietly shapes every lived experience.

CHAPTER 11:
LESSONS FROM ADVANCED CIVILIZATIONS: WHAT HIGHER INTELLIGENCE TEACHES US ABOUT CONSCIOUS EVOLUTION AND LONGEVITY

*"We cannot solve our problems with the same
level of thinking that created them."*
— Albert Einstein

What my soul revealed to me about consciousness across lifetimes did not feel isolated to my journey. As I reflected on Elianore's presence and the vast continuity of awareness she unveiled, I began to sense a larger truth unfolding quietly in the background of human existence. Consciousness is not limited to one planet, one biology, or one civilization. It is a universal principle that appears wherever life becomes coherent enough to perceive itself.

When I Realized Peace Is Higher Intelligence

For as long as I can remember, I carried inside me a deep discomfort with conflict. Growing up in Guayaquil, Ecuador, harsh words and unresolved tension unsettled me more than they seemed to affect others. I did not understand why. I only knew that my nervous system longed for harmony the way lungs long for air. Loud arguments felt unbearable. Injustice pierced me. Even casual unkindness lingered in my heart long after the moment had passed.

For many years, I thought this sensitivity was simply part of my personality. I told myself I was overly emotional, too idealistic, and too gentle for a world that often rewards force. I learned to function. I learned to succeed. I learned to be strong. But beneath all of that, a quiet ache remained every time I witnessed cruelty, division, or unnecessary suffering.

It was not until later in life, after my spiritual awakening deepened, that I began to understand this sensitivity differently. I realized it was not weakness at all. It was recognition. Something inside me remembered a different way of being – a way of existing in which harmony was the natural state, not the exception.

There were moments, especially during periods of deep meditation or long contemplative walks near the ocean, when I would suddenly feel as though I had stepped into a different frequency of existence. In those moments, time felt softer. My body felt lighter. My thoughts became quieter. Within that stillness, I sensed an intelligence that was not personal, not emotional, not human in the ordinary sense – but profoundly loving and exquisitely harmonious.

This intelligence did not feel distant. It felt familiar. I would sit with that feeling and wonder, *What if this is the level of consciousness my soul already knows? What if this is the state from which I once lived?*

As the years passed, this question followed me through my studies of science, spirituality, health, and longevity. The more I learned about coherence, neural regulation, and the impact of emotional states on the body, the more I saw the same pattern everywhere: order sustains life, and chaos depletes it. Peace was not merely a moral virtue. It was a biological and energetic necessity.

One evening, while watching the stars stretch endlessly across the sky, I felt a quiet insight settle into me with certainty: advanced intelligence is not defined by machines, speed, or conquest. It is defined by the capacity to sustain coherence. Any civilization capable of lasting beyond cycles of self-destruction would have had to master its own inner turbulence first.

That realization changed how I viewed both the universe and humanity's future. I began to see that the same principles that govern an evolved civilization must also govern an evolved human nervous system. Fear cannot lead forever. Competition cannot remain the ultimate organizing force. Survival consciousness cannot sustain advanced life. At some point, intelligence must include emotional maturity, ethical coherence, and spiritual integration – or it collapses under its own power.

I recognized this truth not only in theory but in my body. During the most stressful seasons of my life, my health faltered. My energy thinned. My sleep fractured. During the seasons when I rested in trust, clarity, and emotional balance, my vitality returned without struggle. My body mirrored consciousness with absolute fidelity.

It became unmistakably clear: my body was responding less to time and more to coherence. In that understanding, I stopped seeing advanced civilizations as distant, unreachable mysteries. They came into view as inevitable expressions of consciousness that had outgrown fear. Humanity no longer appeared broken but young, brilliant, and powerful, yet still learning to regulate its inner world. What moved me most deeply was the realization that I did not need to wait for some future era.

What moved me most deeply was the realization that I did not need to wait for a future era to live in alignment with higher intelligence. I could practice it now, in my thoughts, in my relationships, in my breath, and in my daily choices. Every time I chose calm over reaction, understanding over judgment, presence over panic, I was participating in the same evolutionary trajectory that shapes civilizations.

In quiet moments, I now feel that I am not only living a

human life; I am contributing to a much larger story of consciousness learning how to inhabit form without violence, without domination, and without fear. And I know now, with certainty, that if higher intelligence exists beyond Earth, it is not foreign to us. It already lives within us.

Mini-Practice: A Moment of Inner Civilization

If you wish, pause for a brief, simple practice. Close your eyes for a few breaths and bring to mind a recent moment of conflict or tension – perhaps in your family, your community, or the wider world. Notice how your body feels as you recall it: your breath, your chest, your shoulders, your jaw.

Now, gently invite a single question into your awareness: *If a truly advanced civilization lived through me in this moment, how would it respond?*

You do not need a perfect answer. Simply notice what softens, what relaxes, or what becomes clearer inside you as you hold this question. Even this small shift is a practice in embodying higher intelligence.

Advanced Civilizations as Mirrors of Potential

For centuries, humanity has looked to the stars with wonder, curiosity, and longing. At first, we sought other worlds through mythology. Later, we searched through telescopes and mathematics. Today, we explore through quantum physics, consciousness research, and a growing understanding that intelligence may not be bound by physical form as we know it.

Across cultures and eras, one truth repeats itself in different languages: life is vast, and intelligence is not exclusive to humanity.

When we speak of advanced civilizations, we are not speaking only of technological superiority. True advancement is not measured by speed, machines, or power over matter. It is measured by coherence of consciousness. A truly advanced civilization must first master harmony within itself before it can master the forces of nature. Without inner coherence, technological progress becomes destructive rather than evolutionary.

This is one of the central lessons higher intelligence offers us: evolution that is not accompanied by consciousness becomes dangerous. History on Earth reflects this truth repeatedly. Every leap in technology has forced humanity to confront its own level of moral and spiritual maturity. When inner development lags behind outer capability, imbalance follows.

If advanced civilizations exist – as many researchers, mystics, and those who report contact experiences suggest – they would necessarily have evolved beyond domination, fear-driven survival, and destructive competition. Their longevity would arise not from control but from alignment.

From a consciousness perspective, longevity is not merely a biological achievement; it is the natural result of living in sustained coherence. On a biological level, coherence expressed through emotional balance, nervous system regulation, and harmonic thought patterns supports cellular repair, slows degeneration, and alters the trajectory of aging itself. Aging shifts from a process of progressive breakdown to a gentler, more adaptive transition.

At the social level, the same coherence reshapes collective life. As emotional regulation and coherent intention increase, violence declines, disease becomes less prevalent, and systems organize around stability rather than crisis. Longevity, then, emerges not as a battle against decline but as an expression of alignment – within the body and across civilization.

In this way, higher intelligence does not only teach us about life beyond Earth. It mirrors what humanity itself is in the process of becoming. The same consciousness that whispered in that quiet communion with my soul is the same consciousness that appears to guide evolution across universes. There is no separation between personal awakening and planetary awakening. The architecture is the same at every scale.

Peace as a Marker of Higher Intelligence

One of the core traits often attributed to advanced civilizations is peace – not peace as a fragile political treaty, but peace as a stable internal state of coherence. This kind of peace arises only when fear no longer governs decision-making and when identity is no longer confined to the survival of the separate self.

In such a state, cooperation replaces competition. Sharing replaces hoarding. Creation replaces domination. Longevity becomes shared rather than hoarded.

Another consistent marker of advanced intelligence is deep respect for life in all its forms. When consciousness expands beyond the limits of egoic identity, life is no longer ranked, exploited, or consumed without awareness. Every form of existence is recognized as an expression of the same universal intelligence. Cruelty becomes inconceivable. Exploitation becomes irrational. The health of the whole becomes inseparable from the health of the individual.

From a biological standpoint, sustained coherence has profound implications. Stress, fear, unresolved trauma, and emotional suppression are among the most powerful accelerators of cellular aging. Advanced civilizations, operating from regulated emotional and mental fields, would naturally experience slower aging, fewer degenerative conditions, and extended lifespans – not solely through medical intervention, but through harmony.

The same principle applies to the human body. When we live in constant survival mode, our cells remain in a state of contraction. In that state, inflammation proliferates, immune resilience weakens, and degenerative processes accelerate. When we live from coherence, safety, emotional integration, and purpose, the nervous system shifts toward repair. The body becomes receptive to regeneration. Longevity becomes less of a struggle and more of a response to alignment.

What advanced civilizations demonstrate is not unreachable perfection, but the natural destination of consciousness when evolution proceeds without interruption by fear.

Humanity at a Crossroads

Humanity currently stands at a crossroads of its own making. We possess extraordinary technological power, yet our emotional and spiritual maturity often lags behind our inventions. We can communicate instantly across the globe, yet many of us struggle to communicate honestly within our families. We can manipulate matter at the atomic level, yet we find it difficult to regulate the thoughts that govern our nervous systems.

This imbalance is not a failure of intelligence. It is an invitation to deepen our consciousness.

Advanced civilizations, whether understood scientifically, symbolically, or spiritually, function as mirrors of what is possible when consciousness leads evolution rather than follows it. They remind us that the destiny of humanity is not endless conflict or inevitable extinction. The destiny of humanity is coherence.

The architecture of awakening within a single soul mirrors the evolution of entire civilizations.

The same movement from fear to awareness, from fragmentation to unity, from contraction to expansion, is visible at every level of existence. What begins in the quiet interior of one human heart ultimately reshapes the destiny of entire worlds.

From this perspective, the work of conscious longevity is not personal alone. It is planetary. Each nervous system that learns peace contributes to collective coherence. Each heart that releases fear strengthens the field of humanity. Each mind that chooses awareness over reactivity gently bends the arc of evolution toward harmony.

Humanity does not need to become something other than itself. It needs to remember what it already is.

The future does not belong to those who dominate

resources or control technology. The future belongs to those who can hold coherent consciousness in an era of acceleration. Longevity in this new era will not be sustained by machines alone. It will be sustained by emotional intelligence, nervous-system mastery, spiritual maturity, and the ability to rest in presence rather than in chronic survival.

At higher levels of intelligence, there is no separation between science and spirit. Physics becomes a language of consciousness. Biology becomes an expression of awareness. Evolution becomes a conscious participation. Longevity becomes the natural outcome of living in alignment with the laws of coherence.

We are not meant to worship higher intelligence. We are meant to grow into it.

Breathing Exercise: Coherence With the Universal Field

(Approximately six minutes.)

If you wish to experience a taste of this coherence in your body, you can explore a simple breath practice.

Sit upright with your spine comfortably aligned and your shoulders relaxed. Allow your hands to rest where they feel most at ease. Begin to inhale slowly through your nose to a gentle count of six, feeling your chest and abdomen expand. At the top of the inhale, pause softly for a count of two, without forcing or straining. Then exhale through your mouth for a slow count of eight, letting your body release tension as the air leaves.

As you inhale, you may silently affirm, "I align with coherence." As you exhale, you might gently repeat, "I release fear and fragmentation." Continue breathing in this rhythm for several minutes, allowing your breath to become like a steady wave. When you feel complete, let your breath return to its natural pattern and notice any subtle changes in your internal state. Your nervous system has just received a lived experience of greater order and ease.

Guided Meditation: Sensing the Greater Intelligence

(Approximately eight to ten minutes.)

To deepen your felt sense of higher intelligence, you may explore this brief meditation.

Close your eyes gently and bring awareness first to your physical body. Feel the support beneath you – the chair, the floor, the ground – and allow your weight to be held. Then begin to notice the space around your body, as if your awareness is gently expanding beyond the outline of your skin.

Sense yourself not only as a body but as a field of perception within a larger field. You do not need to imagine anything elaborate. It is enough to feel that your awareness extends a little beyond your physical form.

When you feel ready, you can ask silently within, "What quality of intelligence is guiding my evolution right now?" There is no need to search for an answer. You are simply inviting a subtle knowing to arise. You may feel a sense of calm, a word, an image, or only a quiet presence. Allow stillness to respond in its own way.

Rest in this awareness for several breaths. Before returning, you might gently affirm, "I am part of a greater coherence." Then bring your attention back to your body, to the room around you, and slowly open your eyes, carrying a trace of that wider intelligence into your next moments.

Reflection Prompts

If you wish to integrate the ideas of this chapter more fully, you may spend some time journaling or contemplating these questions in your own words.

You might explore how your life would change if you trusted that consciousness is evolving through you, and not only around you. You can notice the ways in which fear and coherence alternately shape your health and energy, and how your body responds differently to each state.

You may reflect on what an "advanced civilization of the heart" would look like to you – perhaps in your family, your community, or your country. Consider how your daily emotional state may influence not only your own longevity but the larger field of collective evolution. Finally, you might ask yourself where in your life you are being invited to mature beyond mere survival into coherence, and what small, concrete step could honor that invitation today.

The same intelligence that guides stars, cells, and civilizations breathes quietly within you. Longevity is not a race against time. It is an ongoing conversation with coherence. Humanity's next evolution will not be engineered through force.

It will be remembered through consciousness.

CHAPTER 12:
THE NEW HUMAN: INTEGRATING SOUL, SCIENCE, AND HIGHER CONSCIOUSNESS INTO DAILY LIFE

*"The next evolution of humanity will not be technological alone
— it will be a revolution of consciousness."*

— Maria L. Ellis

The future of human evolution is not waiting for us in distant galaxies or hidden dimensions. It is unfolding quietly in kitchens, workplaces, hospitals, relationships, and ordinary moments of choice. The New Human is not a futuristic species engineered through technology alone. The New Human is a way of being — a synthesis of soul awareness, scientific understanding, and conscious living expressed through everyday life.

The Day My Life Finally Felt Whole

For a long time, my life felt as if it were being lived in compartments. There was the part of me that worked, planned, achieved, and managed everything that needed to be handled. There was the part of me that reflected, prayed, listened inwardly, and sought deeper truth. And there was the part of me that dealt with my body — its energy, its limitations, its needs.

I carried these parts as if they belonged to different versions of me. I moved between them depending on what the day demanded. I did not yet realize how much energy it takes to live disconnected from yourself.

The shift toward wholeness happened quietly. It did not come through a single revelation. It arrived through a growing fatigue with living divided.

One morning, standing in my kitchen as sunlight spilled across the counter, I suddenly felt an unexpected clarity: I no longer wanted to be one person in meditation and another in the world. I no longer wanted to think spiritually but live mechanically. I no longer wanted to care for others with wisdom while silently neglecting myself.

I wanted my life to be one continuous expression of awareness.

That was the day the New Human stopped being an idea for me and became a practice. Integration began with the smallest moments: how I spoke to myself when I made a mistake, how I moved through my day when no one was watching. I noticed how differently my body felt when my thoughts were kind instead of critical, when my pace was gentle instead of rushed, when my actions matched what I claimed to believe.

For the first time in my life, I began to live as if my inner world actually mattered to my physical world.

Science had already taught me that my nervous system, hormones, heart rhythm, and immune response all reacted to perception and meaning. My spiritual life had already taught me that my breath, presence, and awareness shaped the energy of everything I touched. But now I was learning to live as if both were simultaneously true. Something inside me exhaled.

I began to wake in the morning not with urgency, but with curiosity. I would place my hand on my chest and feel my heartbeat before checking the world outside myself. I would ask not only what I needed to accomplish, but how I wished to inhabit the day. Those few quiet seconds changed the tone of everything that followed.

I noticed that when I made decisions from coherence rather than anxiety, my body felt lighter. My digestion improved. My sleep deepened. My resilience expanded. Even my patience with others softened into genuine compassion instead of being forced. I was no longer practicing spirituality in isolation. I was practicing conscious living. Spirituality was no longer something I *visited*; it was something I *lived*. Awareness informed choices, shaped relationships, and guided how energy was spent and restored. Conscious living integrated insight with action, allowing inner understanding to express itself through ordinary life rather than remaining separate from it.

There was a particular afternoon when this integration became undeniable. I had received difficult news that once would have sent me immediately into worry and mental spiraling. I felt the familiar tightening in my chest, the surge of fear in my nervous system.

This time, something different happened. I paused. I breathed. I placed my feet firmly on the floor and felt the support beneath me. I allowed the fear to be present without letting it narrate my future. I softened my shoulders. I stayed. Within minutes, my body began to settle.

The circumstances had not changed – but I had. That was the moment I truly understood what it means to be the New Human. It is not about having fewer challenges. It is about meeting the same challenges with a different internal architecture.

Mini-Practice: A Single Breath of Integration

If you wish, you can feel this shift right now in a simple way. For just a few breaths, let your attention rest on three levels at once: notice your body (its posture, your feet on the floor, your breath moving), notice your thoughts (whatever is passing through your mind), and notice the quiet awareness that is able to witness both. For one inhalation and exhalation, allow all three – body, mind, and awareness

– to be included, without trying to change anything.

That brief moment of inclusion is the essence of integration. Nothing is rejected. Everything is allowed to belong.

Living as One Continuous Field

I began to see how often I had lived as though my body were a tool to be pushed, my emotions something to manage away, and my consciousness something separate from ordinary life. Integration changed all of that.

My body became a partner instead of a project. My emotions became guidance instead of obstacles. My awareness became home instead of a place I visited occasionally.

Even my relationship with time changed. I no longer felt chased by it. I began to feel held within it. I stopped saying, "I don't have time," as often. I started asking, "How present am I with the time I have?" Presence, I discovered, stretched time in ways urgency never could.

I still had responsibilities. I still had deadlines. I still faced uncertainty. But these no longer defined the quality of my existence. They became part of a larger field of meaning instead of the center of it.

Integration also transformed my relationships. I listened differently. I reacted less. I forgave more easily. I stopped needing to be right so often – not because I was trying to be virtuous, but because my nervous system no longer lived in chronic defense. When the inner war softened, outer battles lost their urgency.

I could now see how many years of my life had been shaped by silent survival mode. I could also see how gently and patiently life was now teaching me to live from trust instead of tension.

One evening, after a long but grounded day, I caught my reflection in the mirror. I saw the lines on my face – the evidence of years I had lived, loved, struggled, and grown. Instead of wishing them away, I felt something entirely new: reverence. This face did not signal decline; it represented integration. I was no longer trying to remain young; I was learning how to remain whole.

The New Human, I realized, is not someone who has transcended being human. The New Human is someone who has finally learned how to inhabit being human consciously – with science in the mind, soul in the heart, and awareness in every action.

I no longer lived in separate worlds of faith and fact, spirit and body, inner life and outer life. I lived in one continuous field of meaning. That was the greatest gift of all – not more knowledge, not more control, but more coherence. In that coherence, I felt a kind of vitality no supplement, routine, or strategy had ever given me.

I felt at home inside my own life.

That is when I knew: the New Human is not a distant ideal waiting for the world to catch up. The New Human is born the moment we stop living divided from ourselves. This integration is not theoretical; it is lived.

The New Human as an Integrated Identity

For centuries, humanity separated inner life from outer life. Spirituality was reserved for sacred spaces. Science was confined to laboratories. Daily life unfolded in a third realm governed by habit, urgency, and survival. The New Human dissolves these divisions. Soul, science, and daily behavior become one continuous expression of conscious participation.

This is where conscious longevity becomes real. The New Human does not seek transcendence by escaping life, nor progress by ignoring the soul. The New Human learns how to live awake within the ordinary – how to cook, work, love, grieve, build, rest, and age with awareness. Integration is the defining skill of this new era.

The New Human understands the nervous system while honoring intuition, respects biology while attending to energy, and uses technology without abandoning stillness. This way of being values data and inner knowing equally, integrating what once seemed separate. The New Human does not live in fragments but as a coherent whole.

This integration begins with identity. For most of human history, identity has been constructed primarily through roles: profession, family position, social status, gender expectations, and cultural conditioning. These roles were necessary for survival and social order, but they were never the full truth of who we are.

The New Human lives from a deeper identity: not a fixed self-defined solely by roles, history, or achievement, but a participating field of awareness embodied in time. This identity recognizes the body not as an object to be managed, but as an intelligent interface through which consciousness expresses itself. Thought, emotion, sensation, and intuition are understood as signals within a larger field rather than isolated events.

Living from this perspective changes how one relates to life. Experience is met with curiosity rather than defense, participation rather than control. Time is no longer something to outrun or fear, but a dimension through which growth, learning, and coherence unfold. In this way, identity becomes less about preserving an image and more about staying aligned with the living intelligence moving through each moment.

This does not dissolve personality. It places personality in relationship with the soul. You still have preferences, histories, talents, and limitations. But you are no longer defined solely by them. You become the consciousness that moves through them rather than the structure confined within them.

This identity shift is one of the most powerful regulators of longevity. When identity is fragile and constructed solely around performance, the nervous system remains perpetually vigilant. When identity is grounded in awareness, the nervous system relaxes into coherence. Coherence becomes the baseline from which life is lived.

Breathing Exercise: Integrating the New Human Within

(Approximately five minutes.)

You may wish to explore a brief breath practice that supports this sense of inner integration.

Sit upright with your feet resting comfortably on the floor and your hands either on your thighs or gently over your heart. Allow your spine to lengthen without strain. Begin to inhale slowly through your nose for a count of five, feeling the breath move down into your body. Then exhale slowly through your mouth for a count of seven, allowing your shoulders and jaw to soften as the air leaves.

On each inhale, you may silently repeat the phrase, "I integrate." On each exhale, you might quietly repeat, "I embody." Let your breath remain smooth and unforced, like a gentle tide moving in and out. Stay with this rhythm for several minutes. When you feel ready, allow your breathing to return to its natural pattern and notice how your body and awareness feel together in this moment.

Guided Meditation: Embodying the New Human

(Approximately eight to ten minutes.)

To deepen this sense of integration, you can explore the following meditation.

Close your eyes gently and bring your attention to the natural rhythm of your breathing. Notice the rise and fall of your chest and abdomen. Without effort, allow a soft, steady light to appear in your awareness at the center of your chest. You do not need to see it clearly; it is enough to sense it.

With each inhale, imagine this light expanding gently through your body – through your shoulders, arms, chest, abdomen, legs, and feet – until your whole body feels softly illuminated from within. With each exhale, imagine this same light extending just beyond your body into the space around you, as if your presence is quietly filling your environment with steadiness.

You may wish to silently affirm, "I live as a bridge between soul, science, and daily life." Rest in this sense of embodied wholeness for several breaths, allowing your mind, body, and awareness to rest together in one field of experience.

When you are ready, bring your attention back to the sensations in your body, the weight of your feet on the floor, the contact with your chair, and slowly open your eyes.

Reflection Prompts

If you would like to integrate this chapter more deeply, you may spend some time journaling or reflecting on a few questions.

You might begin by considering the ways in which you are already living as the "New Human" without having named it that way – perhaps in how you care for your body, how you listen to your intuition, or how you bring empathy into your relationships. From there, you can explore where you still feel fragmented rather than integrated, and how those fractures show up in your body, pace, or emotional life.

You may reflect on how your current relationship with work, rest, and connection either supports or erodes your longevity. You might ask what daily life would look like if you treated your nervous system as sacred infrastructure – something to be protected, tended, and honored.

Finally, you may wish to identify one small, concrete shift you could make this week to embody conscious integration more fully. Perhaps it is a morning pause before picking up your phone, a kinder inner voice when you are tired, or a moment of coherent breathing between tasks. Even the smallest change, when repeated with awareness, becomes part of the architecture of the New Human emerging through you.

As the New Human begins to take shape in daily life, a much larger horizon comes into view – the future of our species itself. In the next chapter, we move beyond the individual and into the collective destiny of humanity as we explore **The Future Human: Consciousness, Evolution, and the Next Era of Life on Earth** – how this new level of integration may shape not only personal longevity but the evolutionary direction of our world.

CHAPTER 13:
THE FUTURE HUMAN:
CONSCIOUSNESS, EVOLUTION,
AND THE NEXT ERA OF LIFE ON
EARTH

*"Until you make the unconscious conscious,
it will direct your life and you will call it fate."*

— Carl Jung

The future of humanity will not be shaped by technology alone, nor by biology alone, nor by spiritual aspiration alone. It will be shaped by the integration of all three through consciousness. The Future Human is not merely a more advanced version of the modern individual. The Future Human is a shift in how life itself is understood, inhabited, and stewarded.

The Moment I Realized the Future Was Living Inside Me

For most of my life, I thought of the future as something abstract — something that would arrive later, shaped by forces beyond me, such as technology, politics, economics, and younger generations. I believed the future belonged to those who were coming after me, not to those living it now.

Then, one quiet evening, that belief fell away.

I was sitting alone, reflecting on everything I had been learning about consciousness, healing, intelligence, and longevity. I felt grateful for my awakening, yet a strange sadness drifted beneath that gratitude. The world felt divided, rushed, and afraid. So much advancement, yet so little peace. I found myself wondering whether humanity was truly moving forward – or simply moving faster.

That was when a startling truth arose within me, not as a thought, but as a knowing: The future is not something I will witness. It is something I am already participating in.

That realization changed everything.

I had spent years assuming that my personal awakening was primarily for my healing and growth. In that moment, I understood that every shift I had made within myself – every choice toward coherence, compassion, awareness, and responsibility – was quietly contributing to the larger evolution of humanity.

I was not just living my life. I was shaping the field of consciousness that future lives would be born into. This understanding humbled me deeply.

My daily choices took on new meaning: how I regulated my emotions, spoke in moments of conflict, cared for my body, treated strangers, and talked about fear, aging, technology, and time. None of these were private acts anymore; they were threads woven into the collective future.

The Future Human stopped feeling like a distant species. It felt like a state of being already emerging through ordinary people – through me, through you, through anyone willing to live with awareness.

One afternoon, while watching children play in a park, this truth settled into my body with unexpected force. They moved with such presence, such ease, such curiosity. I thought about the world they would inherit – not only its technologies and climate but its consciousness, including emotional patterns, unhealed wounds, and the accumulated wisdom.

For the first time, I felt my role clearly. I was no longer

just healing my past. I was preparing the future.

My relationship with time shifted again. I stopped feeling as though I were nearing the end of a personal arc. I began to feel as though I stood inside a great relay, holding the baton of consciousness for a brief but meaningful moment before passing it on.

My age no longer felt like a boundary. It felt like a position of stewardship.

I saw how earlier generations had handed the world to me – imperfectly, lovingly, sometimes broken, sometimes inspired. And I realized that I, too, would one day hand the world forward, not only through what I built outwardly but through the quality of consciousness I embodied inwardly.

The Future Human, I realized, is not defined by machines or genetic engineering. The Future Human is defined by how much fear has been transformed into understanding, how much separation into connection, how much raw power into lived wisdom.

And suddenly, the great questions of our time became deeply personal for me: Would we choose speed over presence? Domination over cooperation? Profit over life? Fear over trust?

Or would we finally mature into the deeper intelligence we have always carried within us?

There was a night when this responsibility felt almost overwhelming. The news was filled with conflict, environmental crisis, and technological acceleration. I sat in silence, feeling the weight of it all. For a moment, despair whispered inside me: Are we too late?

Then, just as quietly, another truth answered: It is never too late for consciousness.

Hope returned – not as naïve optimism but as resolve. I came to understand that hope is not the belief that everything will turn out well. Hope is the willingness to show up awake even when the outcome is uncertain.

From that moment on, I stopped waiting for the world to change before living differently. I became the change wherever I stood. I practiced coherence when chaos was easier. I practiced listening when judgment was faster. I practiced calm when fear was contagious. I practiced responsibility when blame felt tempting.

Not because I thought I could save the world, but because I understood that the world is shaped by how each of us inhabits our nervous system and moral choices.

The Future Human began to feel less like a prophecy and more like a quiet daily discipline. The more I lived this way, the more I sensed that humanity's evolution does not advance through dramatic revolutions alone. It advances through thousands of subtle awakenings happening simultaneously across the globe – unseen, uncelebrated, and profoundly transformative.

People choosing kindness over cruelty. Presence over reactivity. Integrity over convenience. Truth over comfort. These are the architects of the future. Somehow, astonishingly, I am one of them.

One morning, standing outside as the sun rose, I felt the warmth on my face and the stillness of the world before it fully awakened. Past and future seemed to dissolve into a single, living now. My breath moved in and out with quiet simplicity.

And I understood: The Future Human is not waiting in tomorrow. The Future Human is being born in this very breath.

I was not too old to shape the future. I was not too small to influence it. I was not separate from it. I was within it.

From that day forward, I stopped asking how much time I had left. I began asking how fully I was willing to inhabit the time that was already mine.

I no longer measured my life by its length alone. I measured it by the depth of awareness I carried, by how much awareness I brought into each interaction, by how much responsibility I took for my inner world, and by how gently I treated the life that moved through me.

The Future Human, I realized, is not a destination we

reach someday. It is a way of being we choose now. And in choosing it, again and again, breath by breath, decision by decision, we quietly shape the next era of life on Earth – not through force, but through consciousness.

Mini-Practice I: Standing in the Relay

If you wish, you can feel this shift in a single, simple moment. The next time you are alone, place your hand over your heart and imagine that all those who came before you are standing behind you, and all those who will come after you are standing before you. For one breath, feel that you are not at the end of anything – you are standing in the middle of a vast relay. Notice how your body feels when you remember that your choices ripple forward.

Mini-Practice II: Becoming the Future Human Today

This short daily practice helps you embody the essence of the Future Human in a way that is simple, grounded, and immediately transformative.

Begin each morning by placing your hand gently over your heart before reaching for your phone or stepping into the day. Take one slow breath and ask yourself, "**What is one way I can live as the Future Human today?**" Allow a single intention to arise – perhaps more patience, deeper listening, conscious breathing, or a moment of genuine presence.

Midday, pause for a brief moment wherever you are. Take three slow breaths and ask yourself, **"Am I living from survival or stewardship right now?"** If you notice tension, urgency, or defensiveness, soften your shoulders, exhale deeply, and choose one small shift that feels coherent with the Future Human you are becoming.

In the evening, before bed, take a final moment of reflection. Ask yourself, **"How did I express the Future Human today, and what did I learn?"** Allow your awareness to honor even the smallest moments of presence or compassion. End with a quiet affirmation: "I am participating in humanity's evolution."

Consciousness as the New Evolutionary Engine

For most of history, evolution was viewed as something that happened to humanity through slow biological adaptation. Today, we stand at a threshold where evolution is becoming something that happens through humanity – consciously, deliberately, and at unprecedented speed. This shift carries enormous promise and profound responsibility.

Consciousness is emerging as the primary driver of the next evolutionary era.

The Future Human will not be defined only by longer lifespans, enhanced intelligence, or technological augmentation. The Future Human will be defined by coherence: alignment between inner life and outer action, between innovation and ethics, between power and wisdom, and between individual expression and planetary responsibility.

Without coherence, advancement fragments. With coherence, advancement becomes evolutionary rather than destructive.

Human history shows that technological intelligence tends to outpace emotional and spiritual maturity. We learn how to build faster than we learn how to steward. We learn how to control before we learn how to care. This imbalance now stands as one of the greatest risks to our species.

The Future Human represents a correction of this imbalance.

This new era is not linear; it is integrative. It does not replace the body with machines or the soul with algorithms. It calls the human being into a deeper partnership with intelligence itself – biological, artificial, planetary, and cosmic. In this partnership, consciousness becomes the regulator.

From Survival to Stewardship

Historically, human evolution was driven by survival. Hunger, threat, disease, and environmental pressure shaped our biology and behavior. The nervous system evolved to detect danger and mobilize quickly. Much of modern life is still governed by this ancient wiring.

But the Future Human will be shaped not by survival alone, but by stewardship.

Stewardship of the body. Stewardship of relationships. Stewardship of technology. Stewardship of Earth.

This shift changes everything about how longevity is understood. Longevity is no longer only about individual preservation. It becomes about the continuity and coherence of life systems. A species cannot extend its life meaningfully while destroying the systems that sustain it.

The Future Human recognizes that personal health, social health, and planetary health are a single, inseparable field.

Evolution by natural selection occurs through random variation and environmental pressure. Conscious evolution occurs through awareness, choice, and integration. The Future Human participates in evolution rather than inheriting it blindly.

This participation does not demand perfection. It requires awareness.

Every time we choose regulation over reactivity, connection over domination, meaning over compulsion, coherence is strengthened at both the personal and collective levels. These micro-choices accumulate into macro-evolution.

The nervous system becomes the primary site of evolutionary training.

A regulated nervous system supports creativity, empathy, long-range thinking, and cooperation. A chronically dysregulated nervous system supports conflict, short-term survival thinking, domination, and fragmentation. The Future Human cannot emerge from unregulated stress alone. It requires a cultural revolution in how safety, presence, and emotional maturity are cultivated.

Long-lived, dysregulated systems collapse. Long-lived, coherent systems flourish.

Technology in the Hands of the Future Human

Technology is neither the savior nor the villain of human evolution. It is an amplifier of whatever level of consciousness currently wields it. The same tools that heal can also harm. The same intelligence that enlightens can also dominate.

The Future Human does not reject technology. The Future Human integrates it with ethical awareness and nervous-system maturity.

Artificial intelligence, genetic engineering, neurotechnology, longevity science, and space exploration will reshape the human experience in ways we cannot yet fully predict. The critical question is not only what we can do but who we are becoming as we do it.

If technology evolves faster than consciousness, humanity's power increases without a corresponding increase in wisdom. This imbalance has repeatedly led to suffering and collapse. If consciousness evolves alongside technology, innovation becomes an expression of care rather than conquest.

The Future Human does not outsource wisdom to machines. The Future Human cultivates wisdom as the governing intelligence behind all tools.

The Evolution of Identity

In earlier eras, identity was shaped primarily by tribe, survival role, and cultural inheritance. In the modern era, identity is largely shaped by profession, performance, and personal narrative. In the future era, identity will increasingly be shaped by the state of consciousness.

People will not identify only by what they do but by how they relate to life. Are they reactive or responsive? Fragmented or integrated? Fear-driven or coherence-centered?

This shift will profoundly alter governance, education, medicine, economics, and family systems. When the state of consciousness becomes as valued as productivity, culture begins to reorganize around regulation, meaning, and wisdom.

The Future Human is not defined by a single culture or ideology. The Future Human is defined by the capacity for conscious relationship across differences.

Longevity in the Next Era

Longevity science will continue to advance rapidly. Cellular rejuvenation, epigenetic reprogramming, regenerative medicine, and precision health will extend human potential lifespan. Yet longevity alone will not guarantee fulfillment.

A long life lived in fragmentation becomes an extended burden. A long life lived in coherence becomes an extended blessing.

The Future Human understands that extended years require expanded meaning. Without meaning, the nervous system deteriorates under the weight of time. With meaning, time becomes a canvas for wisdom.

The next era of longevity will require not only biological repair but existential integration. People will live longer not merely because tissue can be restored but because identity will be rooted in something that does not collapse under change.

When identity is rooted in awareness rather than performance, aging becomes less threatening. As aging becomes less threatening, the chronic stress that accelerates decline softens. The Future Human, therefore, lives longer not only because of medicine but because of how life is interpreted and inhabited.

Planetary Consciousness and Collective Life

Humanity is reaching a stage of development where planetary awareness can no longer be avoided. Climate, ecosystems, oceans, food systems, and biodiversity are no longer background conditions. They are central variables in our survival and evolution.

The Future Human does not see Earth as a resource to be consumed. The Future Human sees Earth as a living partner in evolution.

This partnership requires the maturation of collective consciousness. Exploitation reflects an early stage of awareness. Stewardship reflects a later stage. The shift from one to the other is not primarily technological. It is psychological, emotional, and spiritual.

The Future Human understands that longevity is not personal alone. It is collective. It is ecological. It is intergenerational. A child born today will inherit not only genetic inheritance, but the coherence or fragmentation of the world created by those alive now.

Future societies will face a pivotal choice: govern through fear and control or govern through coherence and participation. Fear-based governance keeps populations in survival mode. Coherence-based governance cultivates long-range thinking, collaboration, and resilience.

The collective nervous system shapes the destiny of a civilization.

Cultures that remain locked in threat perception tend to produce leaders who operate from reactivity and domination. Cultures that cultivate regulation and meaning, by contrast, foster leaders capable of stewardship, humility, and long-term vision.

The Future Human will not overthrow old systems through violence. The Future Human will render old systems obsolete through coherence.

The Spiritual Dimension of the Future Human

As science advances, spirituality is not disappearing. It is evolving.

The future of spirituality will not be confined to institutions or doctrines. It will be expressed through direct experience, embodiment, and integration. The dividing line between sacred and ordinary will continue to dissolve. Daily life will increasingly become the practice. Work will become service. Relationships will become practice. Technology will become stewardship.

The Future Human will not ask only, "What is true?" The Future Human will ask, "What is coherent with life itself?" That coherence becomes the new definition of spiritual maturity.

The Invitation of This Era

Every generation stands at a crossroads, but few stand at one as consequential as this. Humanity now wields tools powerful enough to extend life, alter biology, reshape cognition, and transform the planet itself. The question is not whether change is coming. The question is who we become in the presence of this power.

The Future Human is not guaranteed. It is an invitation.

It is an invitation to evolve not just in what we build, but in who we are. It is an invitation to extend not only lifespan but the depth and reach of understanding we carry through our years. It is an invitation to live not only longer but deeper.

This era will not be defined by a single invention. It will be defined by the maturation of consciousness itself.

You are not a spectator in this evolution. You are a participant.

Every choice you make about how you regulate your nervous system, how you speak in conflict, how you relate to power, how you care for your body, how you honor the Earth, and how you cultivate awareness contributes to the future architecture of humanity.

The Future Human is not born in laboratories or legislated into existence.

The Future Human is realized, one coherent life at a time.

Through that embodiment, the next era of life on Earth begins not with conquest, but with consciousness.

Breathing Exercise: Embodying the Future Human

(Approximately five minutes.)

If you wish to feel this future more tangibly, you can explore a brief breath practice.

Sit upright with your spine naturally aligned and both feet resting on the floor. Place one hand gently over your heart. Inhale slowly through your nose for a count of six, allowing your chest to softly expand. Exhale slowly through your mouth for a count of eight, letting your body soften as the air leaves.

On each inhale, you may silently repeat, "I evolve with awareness." On each exhale, you might quietly repeat, "I steward life with care." Continue this gentle rhythm for several minutes, allowing your breath to deepen and your nervous system to settle. When you are ready, return to your natural breath and notice how your body feels in this moment.

Guided Meditation: Meeting the Future Self

(Approximately eight to ten minutes.)

Close your eyes gently and bring your attention to the natural movement of your breath. Feel the rise and fall of your chest and abdomen.

Now imagine yourself several decades into the future — healthy, coherent, wise, and at peace. You do not need to see every detail. It is enough to sense the quality of this presence. Notice how this future self stands, breathes, and moves through life.

Silently ask within, "What state of consciousness allowed me to become this?" Do not force an answer. Simply allow impressions, feelings, or subtle knowing to arise.

You may wish to affirm quietly, "I am becoming the future I wish to inhabit." Rest with this image and feeling for several breaths. When you are ready, bring your attention back to the sensations of your body, the support beneath you, and slowly open your eyes.

Reflection Prompts

If you would like to integrate this chapter more deeply, you might spend some time journaling or reflecting on a few questions.

You can begin by asking yourself what qualities you believe truly define the Future Human – not only in terms of intelligence or capability but in terms of consciousness, compassion, and coherence. You may explore how your daily choices, habits, and ways of relating contribute to or detract from that future.

You might reflect on the ways in which your nervous system is still trained more for survival than for stewardship and how that training shows up in your reactions, your pace, and your relationship to uncertainty.

You can consider how your understanding of longevity changes when you view it as a collective and planetary responsibility rather than a purely individual goal. Finally, you might ask: What is one small, concrete practice I could begin this week to live more consciously into humanity's future, perhaps a moment of daily coherence breathing, a shift in how you consume news, or a more compassionate way of engaging in difficult conversations?

Even the smallest practice, repeated with awareness, becomes part of the future human story you are already helping to write.

As we look toward the future of humanity, a final and essential question remains: How does healing itself evolve in a quantum universe where energy, intention, and consciousness shape the body at the deepest levels?

In the final chapter of this book, we return to the mystery and science of healing itself as we explore The Quantum Field of Healing: How Energy, Intention, and Consciousness Shape the Body – the frontier where conscious longevity meets the deepest architecture of life.

BONUS CHAPTER A:
YOGA FOR CONSCIOUS LONGEVITY: A PATH OF COHERENCE, PRESENCE, AND CELLULAR RENEWAL

"The body is a vehicle for the soul, and yoga is the path that keeps the engine running smoothly."
— Paramahansa Yogananda

Yoga has long been misunderstood in the modern world as a form of stretching, fitness, or performance. In truth, it is one of the most ancient disciplines of consciousness, a precise method for bringing the body, breath, and awareness into coherence so the deeper intelligence of life can express itself without distortion. At its core, yoga is a relationship practice: a relationship with breath, with sensation, with stillness, and ultimately with the truest self that exists beneath habit and noise. It is a path that does not impose change but reveals it, a process through which the body remembers how to live in harmony with the field that sustains it.

Why Yoga Matters for Longevity

Every true yoga practice, no matter the lineage or style, begins with presence. The moment awareness returns to the breath, the nervous system softens. The moment the nervous system softens, the body shifts from survival to repair. This transition is the essence of longevity. As we have explored throughout this book, what accelerates aging is not time itself, but fragmentation – the gradual separation between mind and body, intention and action, emotion and physiology. When life is lived in a state of chronic disconnection, the nervous system remains strained, repair mechanisms are disrupted, and energy is continually diverted toward managing stress rather than sustaining vitality.

What slows aging is coherence. When thoughts, emotions, behaviors, and biology begin to align, the body receives consistent signals of safety and regulation. Resources shift from defense to repair, from survival to renewal. In this state, aging becomes less about decline and more about adaptation, resilience, and intelligent reorganization over time.

Yoga restores this coherence through gentle but profound mechanisms. Breath regulates the heart's rhythm. Slow movement stabilizes the mind's turbulence. Sustained attention rebuilds neural pathways associated with clarity and emotional balance. Stillness replenishes the energy that modern life continually depletes. Yoga is not simply exercise; it is an environment in which the body can remember safety, reorganize its internal patterns, and return to its natural state of balance. In this way, yoga becomes a quiet medicine that works from the inside out, touching the molecular level through the doorway of awareness.

The True Purpose of Yoga

The original purpose of yoga was never to sculpt a stronger body or achieve extraordinary poses. Its purpose was to refine perception so the practitioner could experience life without distortion, to see clearly, feel deeply, and grow in wisdom. Yoga trains the nervous system to remain steady even when circumstances shift, and this steadiness becomes a source of strength far beyond the practice itself.

True yoga invites the practitioner into intimacy with

their aliveness. Sensation becomes a form of communication. Breath becomes a guide. The mind becomes a servant rather than a tyrant. Over time, yoga dissolves the sense of separation we often feel within ourselves. Body, mind, and awareness begin to move in unified rhythm, and in this unification, vitality increases naturally. Aging becomes softer. Life becomes more spacious. And the self becomes less burdened by tension that was never meant to be carried.

How Yoga Extends Longevity

Yoga supports long life not by force but by reordering the internal environment for healing. When breath deepens, oxygenation improves, inflammation decreases, and the cardiovascular system stabilizes. When emotional tension dissolves through mindful movement, the endocrine system recalibrates, supporting hormonal balance across the lifespan. As mental clutter clears, the brain's capacity for neuroplasticity is strengthened, allowing memory, focus, and creativity to remain vibrant well into older age.

Most importantly, yoga reorients the practitioner toward calm, restorative states in which the body can regenerate more effectively. By decreasing chronic stress signals and increasing parasympathetic activity, yoga slows cellular wear that accelerates aging. It is not a magic pill. It is a daily rebalancing, a consistent reminder that vitality is not created through struggle but through alignment with the body's deepest intelligence.

Yoga as a Field of Coherence

Perhaps the most profound impact of yoga is its ability to harmonize the practitioner with the field of life itself. As breath moves in steady rhythm, the heart's electromagnetic field becomes more coherent. As attention anchors in the present moment, the nervous system relaxes into safety. As awareness becomes spacious, the body begins to reorganize energetically. Yoga, in this way, becomes not simply discipline but a living conversation between the individual and the quantum field of healing.

To practice yoga consciously is to participate in a universal principle: that life flows best where resistance softens, where breath deepens, and where presence returns. In this space, healing becomes possible not through effort, but through allowing.

Yoga as a Lifelong Companion

Yoga is not something we outgrow. It grows with us. It matures as we mature. It softens as we soften. It deepens as awareness deepens. In youth, yoga builds strength. In midlife, it restores balance. In later life, it preserves grace. In every stage, it protects coherence.

I am reminded again and again that yoga teaches the body how to listen, the breath how to guide, the mind how to soften, and the soul how to enter the body without resistance. Nowhere did I understand this more profoundly than in the most painful season of my life when Jenny, my beloved mother, passed away in 2005. My mother's passing left a silence inside me that words could not touch. I missed her in ways that felt physical, as though a part of my body had been taken with her. Grief lived in my chest, heavy and constant. I carried it everywhere, quietly, believing that this pain was simply something I had to endure as the price of love.

At first, I tried to stay strong. I stayed busy. I kept moving. I told myself that time would heal me. But grief does not dissolve through denial. It waits patiently in the body until it is invited to move. It was during this time that I returned to my yoga practice, not as exercise, but as refuge. I did not go to the mat seeking flexibility or strength. I went seeking relief from a sorrow that felt too heavy to hold alone. I moved slowly, often through tears. My breath was shallow at first, trembling with emotion. My body felt fragile, unfamiliar, as if it were learning how to exist without her.

Then, one quiet day during a gentle yoga practice, something changed. I was in a simple resting posture, my breath slow and steady, my palms open. Without effort or intention, tears began to fall. But these tears were different. They were not sharp with anguish. They were soft and releasing. As I surrendered into stillness, I felt something extraordinary: a warm, tender presence moved through me, as real as any physical touch I had ever known.

In that moment, I felt my soul settle fully into my body, not in pain, but in love. It felt as though I was being held from within. The ache in my chest softened. My breath deepened naturally. The grief that had been locked inside me for so long finally found the space to move. I did not push it away. I did not resist it. I allowed it to pass through the field of my body with compassion.

And in that release, something miraculous happened. I felt my mother not as loss, but as love. I realized that holding onto the pain was not honoring her; it kept me stuck in the moment of her departure. Letting go did not mean forgetting. It meant transforming grief into a quieter, gentler connection that could live inside me without breaking my heart.

Through yoga, my body learned how to listen to what my soul had been quietly asking for all along. My breath guided me back into safety. My mind softened its grip on suffering. And my soul entered my body fully to love, to comfort, and to heal me. That was the day I let my mother go – not from my heart, but from my pain. In sorrow, I found peace. In place of anguish, I found acceptance. In place of emptiness, I found a deeper, quieter love. This was not the end of grieving. It was the transformation of grief.

Today, when I practice yoga, I feel her with me – not as absence, but as presence. I now understand that conscious longevity is not only about extending life. It is about learning how to move through love, loss, pain, and healing with awareness and grace – so that nothing hardens us, and nothing closes our hearts.

Yoga gave me back to myself. And through that return, it gave me back my mother in a new and eternal way. This is conscious longevity in motion.

Yoga reminds us that the body is not an obstacle to awakening. It is the instrument of awakening. Through breath, movement, stillness, and awareness, yoga teaches us the most important lesson of all: Longevity is not sustained by force. It is sustained by union. Union with the body. Union with the breath. Union with the present moment. Union with the intelligence that moves through all life.

Breathing Exercise: Longevity Prana Breath

Use this breath to restore energy and coherence at any time of the day.

1. Sit comfortably with your spine upright.
2. Inhale through your nose for a count of four.
3. Hold gently for a count of two.
4. Exhale slowly through your nose for a count of six.
5. Pause for two before the next inhale.
6. Repeat for five to seven minutes.

Silently repeat with each breath, **"I receive life fully. I release with trust."**

Guided Meditation: Yoga as Union

Close your eyes gently. Feel your body resting in stillness.
Notice the quiet intelligence beneath the breath.
With each inhale, feel energy rise gently through the spine.
With each exhale, feel gravity support and stabilize you.
Imagine every cell softening into cooperation.
Imagine your body as a river of slow light.
There is no strain. No striving. No effort to become.
You are already in union.
Rest in this awareness for several minutes.
Before opening your eyes, silently affirm, **"I live in harmony with my body, my breath, and my consciousness."**

Reflection Prompts

1. How has my relationship with my body changed over the years?
2. Where does my body still hold fear, grief, or resistance?
3. How might gentleness transform my approach to health and aging?
4. What would it feel like to practice movement as meditation instead of obligation?
5. How could yoga become a spiritual practice rather than another task?

BONUS CHAPTER B:
CONSCIOUSNESS AS A DAILY PRACTICE: INTEGRATED PATHWAYS TO AWARENESS, HEALTH, AND LONGEVITY

"In the midst of movement and chaos, keep stillness inside of you."
— Deepak Chopra

Emerging research across neuroscience and psycho-physiology suggests that consciousness is not static but a modifiable capacity that influences stress response, cognitive function, and long-term health.

This bonus chapter reflects my ongoing commitment to integrating science, lived experience, and discernment in the exploration of consciousness and longevity. Across my books, I have sought to move beyond fragmented solutions toward a more holistic understanding of human potential across the lifespan. By examining both established frameworks and contemporary practices, my intention is to offer readers practical insight into how consciousness can be cultivated daily, supporting not only a longer life but a more conscious and intentional one.

Consciousness is increasingly understood not as a philosophical abstraction but as a functional and trainable aspect of human experience. Advances in neuroscience, psychoneuroimmunology, and contemplative research have demonstrated that attention, perception, and self-awareness are not passive states. They are dynamic processes shaped through repeated practice, environmental input, and intentional regulation. From this perspective, consciousness becomes both a biological and experiential dimension of longevity.

Across my work on longevity, healthspan, leadership, and purposeful aging, I have emphasized that sustainable well-being arises from alignment between internal awareness and external action. Physical interventions alone – whether nutritional, technological, or pharmaceutical – are insufficient when the nervous system remains chronically dysregulated or attention is perpetually fragmented. Consciousness practices provide the missing bridge, linking inner regulation to outer outcomes in measurable ways.

To understand how consciousness functions as a daily discipline rather than a theoretical concept, it is helpful to examine practitioners who have integrated inner work into complex, high-demand lives over long periods of time. Two such examples, emerging from different traditions yet converging on similar principles, are entrepreneur Jirka Rysavy and physician and consciousness researcher Deepak Chopra.

Rysavy's approach to consciousness is rooted in daily meditation practiced consistently for decades. He has described stillness as foundational to clarity, decision-making, and creative insight. Rather than using meditation reactively, as a response to stress, he treats it proactively as a means of stabilizing attention and reducing cognitive noise before engaging with the demands of leadership and innovation. This emphasis aligns with neuroscientific findings showing that regular meditation alters default mode network activity, enhances attentional control, and improves emotional regulation.

From a physiological standpoint, these effects are particularly relevant to longevity. Chronic stress is a well-documented accelerator of biological aging, contributing to inflammation, metabolic dysfunction, and impaired immune response. By prioritizing daily consciousness practices, individuals like Rysavy create conditions that support autonomic balance and cognitive flexibility – key contributors to long-term vitality.

Complementing this contemporary entrepreneurial model is the more structured and extensively studied framework developed by Deepak Chopra. Chopra's work has played a significant role in bridging Eastern contemplative traditions with Western medicine and scientific inquiry. His approach emphasizes the relationship between consciousness, stress physiology, and self-regulation, framing awareness as a modifiable factor in health and disease.

As a Chopra Certified Health Instructor, I have worked within this framework in both formal and applied capacities. What distinguishes Chopra's methodology is its emphasis on reproducibility and accessibility. Consciousness practices are taught as structured, repeatable techniques designed to regulate the nervous system, improve metabolic balance, and support emotional resilience. These practices are grounded in principles consistent with psychoneuroimmunology and epigenetics, which suggest that perception, meaning, and emotional state influence physiological expression over time.

While the language used by Rysavy and Chopra differs – one emerging from personal experimentation and entrepreneurial inquiry, the other from clinical and educational systems – the behavioral foundations of their practices converge. Both emphasize daily stillness, intentional awareness, and internal coherence. Both treat consciousness not as belief but as discipline. Both demonstrate that sustained inner regulation supports clearer thinking, improved health markers, and a greater sense of purpose.

This convergence is important. It suggests that consciousness practices do not depend on a single explanatory model to be effective. Whether framed through neuroscience, contemplative tradition, or lived experience, the mechanism of change remains consistent: repeated attention training alters baseline functioning. Over time, this shapes perception, stress response, and ultimate behavior.

Throughout my writing on longevity and human development, I return to the principle that awareness precedes choice. Consciousness practices strengthen this awareness, allowing individuals to respond rather than react, to design rather than drift. When practiced consistently, they become a stabilizing force across the lifespan, supporting not only longer life but greater clarity and meaning within that life.

This chapter is not intended to promote any individual, philosophy, or proprietary framework. Instead, it illustrates how consciousness can be operationalized as a daily practice across different contexts. The value lies not in adopting specific language but in committing to consistent inner alignment. Consciousness, when cultivated with discernment and discipline, becomes an essential pillar of longevity.

Converging Paths, Shared Foundations

When viewed together, the practices of Jirka Rysavy and Deepak Chopra reveal an important insight: consciousness operates effectively across diverse frameworks when applied consistently. One path emerges from entrepreneurial experimentation, and the other from structured clinical and educational systems, yet both converge on the same foundational behaviors. Daily stillness, intentional awareness, and internal coherence shape cognitive clarity, physiological regulation, and long-term resilience. This convergence reinforces a central theme throughout my work: consciousness is not a belief system to adopt but a capacity to cultivate.

The Consciousness Practices Model

Across my books, I define consciousness practices as a four-part, integrated model that supports longevity, clarity, and purposeful living. First, awareness involves training attention to observe internal states without judgment. Second, regulation refers to practices that stabilize the nervous system and reduce chronic stress responses. Third, integration ensures that inner awareness informs daily choices, behaviors, and relationships. Finally, consistency transforms isolated practices into lasting traits through repetition over time.

This model allows consciousness to be discussed scientifically, experientially, and practically – without reliance on ideology. It is adaptable across health, leadership, aging, and personal development contexts, making it a unifying framework throughout my work.

In summary, when cultivated through consistent awareness, regulation, and integration, consciousness functions as a stabilizing force that supports cognitive clarity, physiological resilience, and purposeful longevity across the lifespan.

The practices in this chapter are not designed to produce immediate transformation but to establish conditions for long-term change. When consciousness is approached as a disciplined and repeatable practice, it becomes a foundational contributor to resilience, health span, and intentional living.

Breaking Exercise: Interrupting Automatic Patterns of Attention

Before engaging with the practices in this chapter, it is useful to briefly disrupt habitual patterns of attention. Much of human behavior operates on cognitive and physiological autopilot, driven by conditioned responses and environmental cues. This exercise is designed to bring awareness to that baseline state.

Pause for one minute and observe your current mental and physical condition without attempting to change it. Notice the quality of your attention. Is it focused or diffuse? Observe your breathing pattern, your posture, and any areas of physical tension. Simply register these observations as data points. This brief interruption serves as a reset, allowing you to engage the practices that follow with greater clarity and intentionality.

Guided Meditation: Training Awareness and Regulation

This guided meditation is designed to support two core elements of the Consciousness Practices Model: awareness and regulation. The intention is not to induce a particular state but to train attention and stabilize the nervous system through simple, repeatable steps.

Begin by sitting comfortably with your spine upright and your feet grounded. Allow your eyes to close or soften your gaze. Bring your attention to your breath without altering its rhythm. Notice the sensation of air moving in and out of the body.

As thoughts arise, acknowledge them without engagement and gently return your attention to the breath. This process reflects a fundamental principle of attentional training: redirection without judgment. Over time, this practice strengthens cognitive flexibility and reduces reactivity.

Next, bring awareness to your body. Notice any areas of tension and allow them to soften with each exhalation. This step supports autonomic regulation, shifting the nervous system toward balance. Remain in this state of attentive observation for several minutes, maintaining a relaxed yet alert posture.

Before concluding, set a simple intention for the remainder of your day. This intention should be practical and observable, such as responding more deliberately to stress or pausing before making decisions. Gently return your attention to your surroundings and open your eyes when ready.

Reflection Prompts: Integrating Consciousness into Daily Life

Reflection is essential for integration, transforming isolated practices into lasting behavioral change. The following prompts are designed to help you connect the awareness gained during this chapter to your daily experience.

Consider how your baseline state of attention influences your health, decision-making, and relationships. In what situations do you notice the greatest loss of awareness or regulation? Reflect on how consistent consciousness practices might alter your response in those moments.

Examine your current routines. Where could brief periods of intentional stillness be realistically integrated into your day? Identify one practice from this chapter that you are willing to repeat consistently over the next week.

Finally, reflect on the role of consciousness in your broader life goals. How might greater internal coherence support not only longevity but also clarity of purpose and quality of engagement with others? These reflections are not meant to be answered once but revisited as your practice evolves.

APPENDIX:
YOGA PRACTICE GUIDE
FOR CONSCIOUS LONGEVITY

A Weekly Schedule for Body, Breath, and Awakening

This Yoga Practice Guide is designed to support **life-long vitality, nervous-system balance, emotional integration, and higher awareness**. These weekly schedules honor the natural rhythms of the body and are intentionally gentle, restorative, and sustainable.

You may follow them exactly as written or modify them according to your health, energy, and physical condition. Consistency matters more than intensity.

Each session includes:

- Gentle movement (Asana)
- Conscious breath (Pranayama)
- Rest or meditation (Integration)

Always listen to your body. Discomfort is a signal to soften, not push.

Weekly Schedule 1: Beginner and Restorative Longevity Practice

(Ideal for beginners, seniors, chronic fatigue, recovery, or high stress.)

(Twenty to thirty minutes per day.)

Monday: Gentle Spine and Breath

- Seated spinal movements (five minutes)
- Neck, shoulders, wrists, ankles (five minutes)
- Longevity Prana Breath (five minutes)
- Short seated meditation (five to ten minutes)

Tuesday: Restorative Lower Body

- Gentle hip circles
- Seated forward fold
- Supported recline or legs up the wall
- Slow breath and body scan

Wednesday: Nervous System Reset

- Chair yoga or floor stretching
- Long exhalation breathing
- Guided relaxation or Yoga Nidra

Thursday: Heart and Chest Opening

- Gentle heart-opening postures
- Shoulder rolls
- Compassion breath
- Gratitude meditation

Friday: Balance and Coordination

- Seated or standing balance work
- Slow, mindful transitions
- Coherence breathing

Saturday: Full Body Restorative

- Supported restorative poses
- Long holds with bolsters or pillows

- Silent rest

Sunday: Integration and Reflection

- Very gentle stretching
- Guided meditation
- Journaling or reflection

Weekly Schedule 2: Intermediate Conscious Longevity Practice

(For those with some yoga experience.)

(Thirty-five to forty-five minutes per day.)

Monday: Spine and Energy Flow

- Gentle Slow Flow (Vinyasa-based, low intensity)
- Seated and standing spinal flexion and extension
- Prana Flow Breathing
- Seated Mindfulness Meditation

Tuesday: Strength with Softness

- Standing Hatha yoga poses with chair support
- Gentle core activation (supine or seated Pilates-style support)
- Extended restorative relaxation

Wednesday: Restorative Healing Day

- Yin Yoga or Restorative Yoga
- Diaphragmatic deep breathing
- Yoga Nidra (Guided Yogic Sleep)

Thursday: Heart–Brain Coherence

- Heart-opening Hatha poses and gentle balance work
- Heart-focused coherence breathing

- Coherence or loving-kindness meditation

Friday: Fascia and Joint Health

- Myofascial release yoga or slow mobility yoga
- Gentle full-body stretching
- Quiet rest in Savasana

Saturday: Flow and Stillness

- Gentle Vinyasa flow or slow Hatha home practice
- Long Savasana
- Breath anchoring meditation

Sunday: Spiritual Integration

- Seated meditation practice
- Slow Pranayama (Nadi Shodhana or Extended Exhale)
- Reflective journaling or contemplative prayer

Weekly Schedule 3: Advanced Conscious Longevity Practice

(For long-time practitioners or those in strong physical condition.)
(Forty-five to sixty minutes per day.)

Monday: Energy Activation

- Dynamic Slow Vinyasa Flow (moderate intensity)
- Spinal Mobility and Strength Work (flexion, extension, rotation)
- Gentle Breath Retention (Kumbhaka-Light)
- Seated Awareness Meditation

Tuesday: Strength and Balance

- Standing Hatha Yoga Series (Warrior poses, balance postures)

- Core and Leg Strengthening (functional yoga conditioning)
- Extended Savasana (Final Relaxation)

Wednesday: Deep Restoration

- Yin Yoga and Restorative Yoga
- Nervous-System Reset Breathing (long exhale, vagal toning)
- Guided Meditation or Yoga Nidra

Thursday: Heart and Consciousness

- Heart-Opening Hatha Sequence (gentle backbends, chest openers)
- Heart–Brain Coherence Breathing
- Awareness or Loving-Kindness Meditation

Friday: Mobility and Longevity Joints

- Joint-Focused Mobility Yoga (hips, knees, shoulders, spine)
- Myofascial Release and Fascia Hydration Yoga
- Gentle Breathwork for Circulation

Saturday: Integrated Practice

- Mixed Hatha–Vinyasa Flow and Restorative Integration
- Extended Meditation Practice (twenty to thirty minutes)

Sunday: Silence and Reflection

- Minimal Movement or Gentle Stretching
- Extended Seated Meditation or Silent Sitting
- Reflective Journaling or Contemplative Prayer

Daily Time-Limited Practice (For Busy Days)

Even on your busiest days, aim for **ten minutes minimum**:

- Three minutes of slow breathing
- Four minutes of gentle stretching
- Three minutes of stillness

Longevity is preserved through **consistency, not perfection**.

Breath-Focused Emergency Reset

(Any time, anywhere.)

When stress spikes:

1. Inhale for four counts
2. Exhale for six counts
3. Repeat eight to ten rounds
4. Relax jaw and shoulders
5. This instantly activates repair mode in the nervous system.

Seasonal Adjustments for Longevity

Longevity is not sustained through rigid routines alone; it is preserved through rhythm, responsiveness, and harmony with the natural cycles of life. The body is not separate from nature; it is an extension of nature's intelligence. Just as the Earth moves through seasons of growth, peak energy, transition, and rest, so too must the human body be supported differently throughout the year. Yoga practiced in alignment with the seasons deepens coherence between the body, the nervous system, and the universal field, allowing vitality to be renewed rather than depleted.

Spring: Gentle Detox, Twists, and New Beginnings

Spring is the season of renewal, emergence, and upward-moving energy. After the stillness and heaviness of winter, the body naturally seeks to clear stagnation and awaken circulation. Gentle detoxifying yoga sequences in spring emphasize twisting postures that massage the internal organs, stimulate digestion, and support the liver's natural detoxification processes. Practices during this season should feel light, fluid, and expansive, encouraging both physical and emotional release. Spring is also a time for new intentions, making it ideal for breathwork that energizes the nervous system without strain and for meditation practices focused on growth, clarity, and fresh direction.

Summer: Circulation Work and Cooling Breath

Summer carries the height of yang energy, expansion, warmth, activity, and outward expression. During this season, the focus of yoga shifts toward supporting healthy circulation, protecting the heart, and preventing overheating of the nervous system. Gentle flowing sequences enhance blood and lymphatic movement without excessive intensity. Cooling breath techniques, such as longer exhales or soft nasal breathing, help regulate body temperature, calm excess fire, and maintain emotional balance. Summer practice should cultivate joy and openness while also honoring the body's need for moderation and hydration.

Autumn: Lung and Immune Support with Grounding Practices

Autumn is the season of transition, contraction, and preparation for rest. As the external environment cools and daylight shortens, the body naturally turns inward. Yoga for autumn emphasizes grounding, stability, and immune fortification. Practices that gently open the chest and strengthen the respiratory system support lung health and protect against seasonal vulnerabilities. Slower, rooted postures stabilize the nervous system and help release grief and emotional residue often associated with this transitional season. Autumn is also a powerful time for letting go of physical tension, emotional burdens, and habits that no longer serve the next cycle of life.

Winter: Restorative Yoga, Deep Restoration, and Longer Sleep

Winter is the season of stillness, introspection, and deep regeneration. Nature withdraws into quiet restoration, and the human body is designed to do the same. Yoga during winter should emphasize restorative poses, long holds, gentle stretching, and extended periods of rest. The nervous system naturally gravitates toward repair mode during this season, making winter an ideal time for Yoga Nidra, breath-based meditation, and self-healing practices. Longer sleep, reduced stimulation, and more inwardly focused awareness support cellular repair, immune resilience, and hormonal balance. Winter is not a time for force or intensity; it is a sacred season of renewal where longevity is built through rest rather than effort.

By honoring these seasonal adjustments, yoga becomes not just a daily practice but a living dialogue with nature itself. Longevity is preserved not by resisting the seasons but by moving with them – allowing the body, the breath, and consciousness to remain in rhythm with the cycles that sustain all life.

Safety and Medical Considerations

Always consult your physician before beginning a yoga practice if you have a heart condition, have recently undergone surgery, experience severe joint issues, are in a high-risk pregnancy, or have neurological disorders, as yoga should always support healing and never place undue strain on the body.

How to Measure Progress in Conscious Longevity Yoga

Progress is not measured by how flexible you become or how advanced your poses appear, but by better sleep, calmer reactions to stress, reduced pain or inflammation, improved mood, an increased sense of peace, and greater embodiment and presence – these are the true biomarkers of longevity.

Final Teaching of the Yoga Appendix

Yoga is not something you do to your body; it is something you do with your consciousness. Over time, yoga will not only change how your body moves – it will change:

How your nervous system responds to life

- How your emotions rise and fall
- How your mind softens
- How your spirit inhabits your form

And this is the deepest promise of yoga: You do not practice yoga to become flexible.

You practice yoga so life can move through you without obstruction.

ACKNOWLEDGMENTS

This book emerged from a long arc of curiosity, reflection, and lived experience. While the ideas presented here are my own, they were shaped by a wide constellation of thinkers, teachers, conversations, and moments of stillness that made inquiry possible.

I am deeply grateful to the scholars, philosophers, scientists, and futurists whose work continues to expand our understanding of consciousness, complexity, and human potential. Their willingness to explore questions that do not yield easy answers has provided both foundation and inspiration for this work. In particular, I acknowledge the intellectual lineage that bridges philosophy, neuroscience, systems theory, and contemplative traditions, reminding us that knowledge advances most meaningfully when disciplines remain in dialogue.

I extend my appreciation to the researchers and practitioners who labor at the edges of what is known — those who challenge reductionist assumptions and invite more integrative models of mind, awareness, and reality. Their courage to ask why as persistently as how has influenced the spirit of this book.

My gratitude also goes to the many individuals — friends, colleagues, students, and fellow seekers — whose questions, insights, and lived experiences quietly informed these pages. Consciousness is not studied in isolation; it is revealed through relationship, reflection, and the shared human condition. Every thoughtful conversation and moment of attentive listening contributed in ways both visible and unseen.

I am especially thankful for the periods of silence, contemplation, and inner inquiry that allowed these ideas to take shape. In a world increasingly defined by speed and stimulation, the discipline of slowing down remains essential to any genuine exploration of awareness.

Finally, I acknowledge my family, whose presence and patience created the space for this work to unfold. Their support – often expressed simply through understanding – was indispensable.

If this book succeeds in inviting deeper reflection, ethical consideration, or a renewed sense of shared responsibility for our collective future, it is because it stands on the shoulders of many – known and unknown – who continue to illuminate the evolving landscape of human consciousness.

ABOUT THE AUTHOR

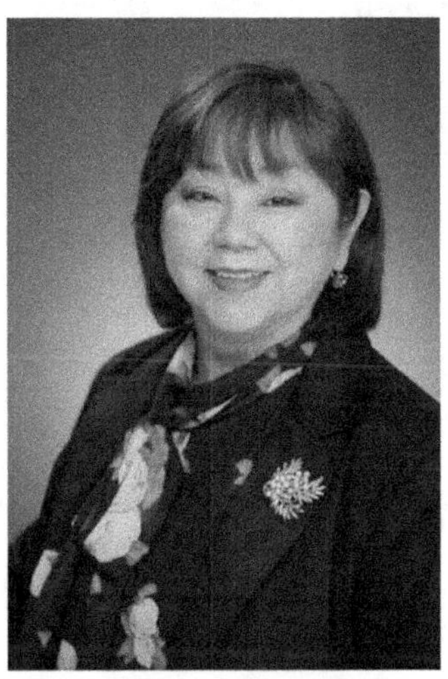

Maria L. Ellis, BBA, MBA, is a seasoned investor, business leader, and educator with a deep passion for helping others build lasting wealth through real estate. With decades of experience spanning finance, entrepreneurship, and strategic investing, Maria has mentored countless individuals to take control of their financial futures and invest with clarity, confidence, and purpose.

She is the founder of a family real estate investment firm, where she and her team acquire, manage, and grow multi-family portfolios across thriving U.S. markets. Known for her practical wisdom, compassionate leadership, and values-based approach, Maria believes that real estate is not just about properties – it's about people, impact, and legacy.

Maria is also a published author of multiple books on entrepreneurship, wellness, longevity, and women's empowerment. Her writing reflects her life's mission: to educate, inspire, and empower others to live fully and invest wisely.

When she's not negotiating deals or guiding investors, Maria enjoys traveling with her family, mentoring the next generation, and living a purpose-driven life filled with service, joy, and growth.

Connect with Maria
Email: <u>mellis@fsacap.com</u>
Mobile: 973-216-4181

ABOUT ELLIS PUBLISHING HOUSE

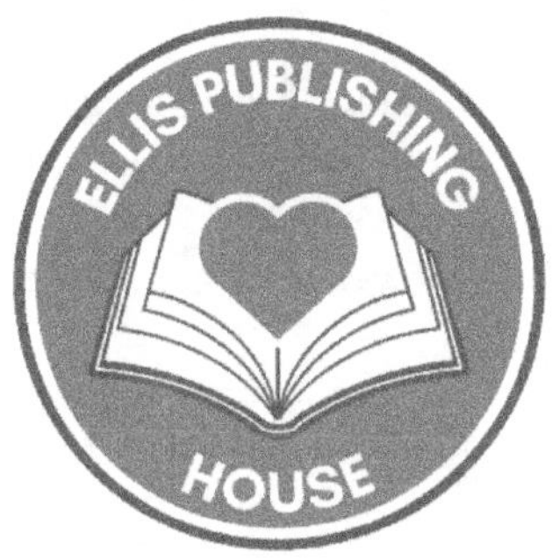

Ellis Publishing House presents the work and vision of bestselling author and educator Maria L. Ellis, BBA, MBA. Founded to bring clear, useful ideas to a wide readership, the imprint focuses on practical nonfiction with enduring value – finance and business, health and longevity, leadership, caregiving, real estate, and poetry – alongside the signature *Journey to Wellness, Freedom, and Legacy* series. Editions are available in English and Spanish across print, eBook, and audio.

Maria's career spans international banking, investment advising, and financial planning, experience that informs her grounded approach to money, leadership, and long-term well-being. A graduate of the Harvard Business School Owner/President Management program, she holds business degrees from the University of Massachusetts Amherst and has served in leadership and advisory roles across education and nonprofit boards. Her books and talks emphasize clarity, compassion, and action – helping readers make better decisions for themselves, their families, and their communities.

Ellis Publishing House exists to advance that mission: books that translate expertise into everyday tools, invite thoughtful reflection, and encourage readers to build not only success but also significance. The catalog includes guides to financial freedom, family business legacy planning, entrepreneurial health, longevity, real-estate investing, leadership, caregiving, and a poetry collection that celebrates life on earth.

In all of its publishing, Ellis Publishing House favors ideas with measurable impact, stories with heart, and designs made to last — work shaped by Maria L. Ellis's commitment to service, integrity, and accessible excellence.

OTHER BOOKS BY MARIA L. ELLIS, BBA, MBA

Achieve Financial Freedom: The Road Map to Financial Success

Family Business Legacy Plan: The Ultimate Guide to Creating a Legacy for Your Family without Paying too Much in Taxes

Redefining Entrepreneurial Success: A Guide to a Healthy and Holistic Lifestyle

Longevity: Reinvent Yourself at Any Age

Life on Earth: Poetic Perspectives

Golf: A Course in Business: A Few Lessons Golf Can Teach Us About Management & Entrepreneurship

From Operator to Entrepreneur: Unlocking the Power of Visionary Leadership

Stolen Memories: A Journey Through Alzheimer's

Designing Your Longevity: A Personalized Blueprint for Thriving Longer with Energy, Purpose, and Vitality

Investing in Multifamily Real Estate: A Guide to Investing for Income, Impact, and Generational Wealth

Beyond Barriers: Women's Progress from Mid-Twentieth Century to Today

Life on Earth, Volume II: Poems That Inspire and Empower Women and Girls

www.ingramcontent.com/pod-product-compliance
Lightning Source LLC
Chambersburg PA
CBHW051508050726
47594CB00010B/4013

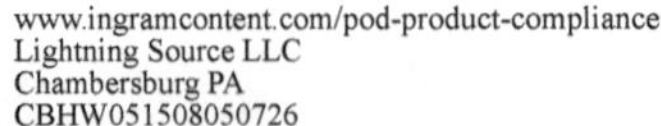